DON'T
PANIC
THIRD EDITION

REID WILSON, Ph.D.

DON'T
PANIC

THIRD EDITION

Taking Control
of Anxiety Attacks

HARPER

NEW YORK · LONDON · TORONTO · SYDNEY

HARPER

HarperCollins books may be purchased for educational, business, or sales promotional use. For information, please write: Special Markets Department, HarperCollins Publishers, 10 East 53rd Street, New York, NY 10022.

Library of Congress Cataloging-in-Publication Data

Wilson, Robert R. (Robert Reid)
   Don't panic : taking control of anxiety attacks / by Reid Wilson.—3rd ed.
     p. cm.
   Includes index.
   ISBN 978-0-06-158244-8
   1. Panic attacks. 2. Anxiety. 3. Self-help techniques. I. Title.
   RC531.W48 2009
   616.85'22—dc22   2008021968

   11 12 13 OV/RRD 10 9 8 7 6 5

To

brother Phill Wilson and

sister Karen Ann Christenbery

Contents

Part I
Identifying the Problem

Part II
The Nature of Anxiety Attacks

Part III
Don't Panic *Live*:
Your Moment-by-Moment Strategies

Part IV
Support When You Need It

Acknowledgments

Pursuing a career in clinical psychology fulfills two of my most cherished lifelong dreams: to continually explore the world of ideas as an eager and naive student and simultaneously to give to others in a way that makes a difference. This book is a reflection of a lifetime of learning, and I hope it in some small way honors those who have nourished and inspired me. Theoretically, it is a synthesis of the work of hundreds of dedicated professionals in a surprisingly broad spectrum of fields. I had planned to acknowledge every gifted professional I have had the honor of directly studying or working with in the fields of anxiety, strategic and paradoxical treatment, and positive psychology. After thirty-five years of being powerfully influenced by the work of others, the list grew to 140, and I surrendered to the page limits granted me here. I am humbled by the gifts of my teachers throughout my professional life.

Rich Simon, PhD, personally guided my writing style in such a way that I have returned to the excitement of being a writer after ten years of frustration. Jeff Sapyta, PhD, synthesized the newest research in the field with skill and adeptness. My "clean team" of Ginger Gialanella, MS, Joanna Wilson,

BFA, Mike Gialanella, MS, Camille Bell, RN, and Brian Leahy, BFA, commented on the readability of all my new chapters. John Ware, my agent and friend, always offers just the right support. And the baristas at Open Eye Café—with its assorted music, children, runners and bikers, discussions and banter—kept me focused and happy throughout this year.

I have long felt the care of my Ericksonian friends, Michael Yapko, PhD, Stephen Lankton, MSW, and Jeffrey Zeig, PhD, and my closest buddies in the anxiety field, Jim Wilson, MA, Sally Winston, PsyD, and Marty Seif, PhD. My friends and colleagues at the Anxiety Disorders Treatment Center—Annette Perot, PhD, and Julie Pike, PhD—inspire me with their creativity. Sylvia Lloyd keeps me on schedule and stays on top of all the office technology. I am grateful to the staff of the Countway Library at Harvard University Medical School and the Health Sciences Library at the University of North Carolina for the use of their valuable resources.

My four lifelong friends—William "Bud" Garrison, Alan Konell, Bruce Buley, and Frank Cole—have joined me in adventures that have opened my heart, expanded my perception of the potential of life, and given me the gift of self-love. Robert and Ann Wilson have long been my steadfast, loving supporters. Bentha Wilson continues to inspire me with her extraordinary blend of optimism, generosity, and assertiveness. Patrick and Joanna Wilson, I'm happy to say, love me always.

Reid Wilson, Ph.D.
Chapel Hill, North Carolina
June 2008

Foreword

Panic sufferers—hope is on the way. In this new and updated edition of *Don't Panic*, Dr. Wilson explains why you suffer from this debilitating form of anxiety and precisely what you need to do to recover from it. He has drawn from both the latest research on panic and his vast experience successfully working with panic patients to develop a protocol that works. And he teaches you how to implement this effective program, step-by-step.

Panic attacks can be intensely frightening and demoralizing. In the midst of one, you may believe that you are about to die, lose control, go crazy, or experience another catastrophic outcome. Even though you may have had dozens or even hundreds of panic attacks, and find that the catastrophe you fear never comes true, why, then, do you still fear panic? As Dr. Wilson explains, you have maladaptive (unhelpful) attitudes and behaviors that keep the disorder going. You are sure, despite all evidence to the contrary, that the *next* time a catastrophe is highly likely to happen. So you avoid experiences that may provoke panic, and when you can't, you do what you can to diminish your panic symptoms. In this way, you never learn that while panic can feel intensely distressing (both physiologically and psychologically), it simply isn't dangerous (absent an extremely serious medical condition such as chronic obstructive pulmonary disease).

Dr. Wilson's book will help to dispel the fear and confusion that accompany panic attacks. In Part 1, you learn what a panic attack is, why you experience intense and rapid physiological changes, and how to differentiate panic from organic conditions. Dr. Wilson describes the similarities and differences between panic and other anxiety disorders. He also demonstrates the power of beliefs about oneself, and how earlier experiences can lead you to feel helpless, vulnerable, self-critical, and dependent on others—which sets the stage for the development of panic disorder.

In Part 2, Dr. Wilson describes how panic undermines your confidence, seeming, at first, to strike out of the blue. Because you don't know when you will experience another attack, you remain constantly on guard. But you will learn that panic does not just occur spontaneously. Panic attacks are always preceded by your *thinking*. If you notice a change in your body or mind, and catastrophize about it ("Oh, no! This is terrible! What if I lose control!"), you will feel highly anxious. If you then focus on your anxiety symptoms, they can increase in intensity until they reach a level of panic. Over time, you start to dread situations in which you have previously experienced panic. You think about entering a feared situation, anticipate a negative outcome, and doubt your ability to handle the consequences. You feel anxious. Then, you decide either to avoid the situation altogether or to enter the situation but do whatever you can to diminish your physiological arousal. *You never learn that even if your symptoms intensify, the catastrophe you fear still would not happen.* So when you begin to feel panicky, your body and mind go into full-fledged emergency mode. Dr. Wilson teaches you how to override your "emergency response" by changing your interpretation of your symptoms and modifying your behavior.

Part 3 teaches you how to adopt a new attitude toward panic. Instead of prolonging your panic disorder by fearing panic, fighting against panic attacks, trying always to avoid panic, and worrying about the recurrence of panic, you will learn how to (1) seek out opportunities to practice facing situations you fear, (2) envision coping with the consequences you fear, (3) modify your tendency to focus on unrealistic consequences, (4) allow yourself to experience panic symptoms without fighting them, (5) reduce your vigilance of symptoms, (6) tolerate uncertainty, and (7) accept the experience of panic and anxiety. Through repeated practice, you will see the value of wanting to feel discomfort and uncertainty so you can prove to yourself that panic, while highly distressing, is not dangerous and that you can handle whatever arises. You will gain a sense of self-confidence and self-efficacy, a cornerstone of independent functioning.

If you are not yet ready to face your fears, Part 4 teaches you a step-by-step process to build skills, support, and confidence. You will learn the "Calming Response" to release tension and relax your body and mind, through breathing exercises, relaxation exercises, and meditation. You will set short-term goals and tackle small challenges one at a time, keeping your focus on the task at hand instead of looking at additional challenges ahead. You will learn to observe your mind, gaining distance from your negative thoughts which will allow you to slow down and quiet your fears. Then you will develop a supportive, helpful internal voice to deal with the worried, hopeless, and self-critical messages of your mind and to aid you in your efforts to confront panic. A final chapter provides important information about possible medications, their indications and side effects, and guidance to judge whether medication might be beneficial for you.

We believe that you will find *Don't Panic* to be valuable and empowering. You will understand what panic is, why it strikes, and what you can do to recover and regain your life.

Judith S. Beck, Ph.D.
Clinical Associate Professor of Psychology in Psychiatry
University of Pennsylvania
Director, Beck Institute for Cognitive Therapy and Research

Aaron T. Beck, M.D.
University Professor of Psychiatry
University of Pennsylvania
President, Beck Institute for Cognitive Therapy and Research

Identifying

PART I

the Problem

CHAPTER 1

Introduction:
The Panic Attack

It is as though the symptoms jump you from behind. With little warning the heart begins its rapid pumping, a cold perspiration beads the forehead, trembling hands want to hide from view. The throat attempts in vain to swallow as any moisture remaining in the mouth disappears.

Your mind races to retain some semblance of control. "Just relax! Stay calm!" is the silent command. But you place little faith in such words. And why should you? They have always failed to relieve the anarchy of the body in the past.

The more you grip to keep control, the less control you feel. Panic! Seconds pass like minutes as your mind is pulled in two directions. First, to the past: "This is like last month, when I became so weak that I almost fainted." Then, to the body with a mind of its own: "I can't catch my breath. I'm trying. I can't!" The future rushes to the present: "What if this keeps up? I could pass out. If my heart beats any faster I could have a heart attack."

At that moment the fear of humiliation crowds the noise of the mind. "Everyone's going to see me collapse. I've got to get out of here." With the same suddenness that this attack started, you make your escape out of the door of the conference room or the movie theater, the doctor's office or the grocery store. The farther you get from the scene, the more comfortable you feel.

This scenario is what I call *the moment of panic:* an internal experience, supported by physical sensations, that you have suddenly and dangerously lost control of your circumstances. The changes in the body and mind take place so rapidly and unconsciously that you experience them as an "attack" of panic or anxiety.

All of us have experienced the physical sensations of anxiety. We get butterflies in the stomach before we give a speech or sore, tense muscles after driving for an hour through a rainstorm. But the experience of general anxiety is quite distinct from the overwhelming sensations of a panic attack.

An example may clarify the difference. Have you ever faced a physical emergency alone, one that you were ill prepared to handle? Imagine opening your cellar door to the sound of water splashing onto the concrete floor. You run down the stairs, half guided by your feet, half carried by your arms pushing off the handrails. How fast do you size up the situation? How many options do you rule out in the first thirty seconds? "Can I stop it with my hand? No . . . How about tying it with a rag? Is there a rag around? Won't work! Where's this pipe coming from? Where's the main valve?" Your eyes move rapidly, absorbing every detail that might play a role in reducing the damage caused in the flooding basement. "Grandma's chest of drawers, it's getting ruined! Should I move it? Stop the water first. Where is that valve?! There's the trash can. No use, the water's spraying too broadly. Who can I call?"

If you freeze the action of the scene at this precise moment, you would recognize in yourself many of the physical sensations found in what we call a panic attack. The muscles are tense, ready to respond immediately to any directions from the brain ("Get down those stairs—*now!*"). The blood is rushing to the brain to stimulate the thought processes. The heart and the respiration rates both rapidly increase to produce the shifting of blood throughout the body, a process essential to energetic action.

Each of us should be thankful for the incredible ability of our mind to instantly and automatically respond in such an emergency. How many of us have been saved from injury or death on the highway because our right foot slammed on the brake while our hands pulled on the steering wheel—all this before we had time even to think the command, "Watch out for that car!"

Brilliant as this built-in emergency system is, sometimes things can go awry. During panic, the body responds with many of the same physical changes that take place during an emergency. However, panic is an exaggeration of our emergency response. Instead of taking advantage of the body's rapidly increased strength, we become overwhelmed by a variety of physical sensations. The more we focus our attention on these internal changes, the more anxious we become and the less able we are to reassure ourselves.

A panic attack—also called an "anxiety attack"—causes the fastest and most complex reaction known within the human body. It immediately alters the functioning of the eyes, several major glands, the brain, heart, lungs, stomach, intestines, pancreas, kidneys, and bladder and the major muscle groups. Within the cardiovascular system, the heart increases its rate of contractions, the amount of blood it pumps with each contraction, and the pressure it exerts as blood is pumped into the arteries. The vessels that channel blood into the vital organs and skeletal muscles expand, increasing their blood flow, while the blood vessels in the arms, legs, and other less vital parts of the body begin to constrict, reducing blood flow in those areas.

While this is taking place, your rate of respiration increases. The pupils dilate to improve distance vision. Within the gastrointestinal system, all digestive activity is diminished. As a result, your metabolism that converts food into energy is enhanced, and increased amounts of sugars and fatty acids are secreted into the bloodstream.

Your subjective experience during a panic attack can vary greatly. Certain reactions (such as noticing your heart rate) are directly related to the physiological changes I have just mentioned. Others (such as the fear that you are dying) are produced by your mental and emotional responses to these sensations. Generally speaking, the more reactions you have during the attack and the greater the intensity of each reaction, the more devastated you feel by this assault. Here are some common sensations:

- *The head.* Decreased blood flow to the brain, caused by hyperventilation, may lead you to feel lightheaded or dizzy, as though your head is "swimming." You may feel faint.
- *The body.* You begin to perspire, have hot and cold flashes, feel numb or experience prickling or tingling. You feel as though you are whirling about (the sensation of vertigo). The whole body feels fatigued or depleted.
- *The mind.* You feel disoriented, confused or unable to concentrate. You feel cut off or far away from your surroundings (called derealization). Your body can feel unreal, as though you are in a dream (called depersonalization). You become irritable or short-tempered. Common fears are of fainting, going crazy, having a heart attack, dying, making a scene or becoming trapped.
- *The eyes.* Your eyes flicker or twitch. You may have difficulty focusing on objects, or they might appear blurry.

Figures such as numbers on a page "jump around" or appear reversed.

- *The mouth and throat.* Your mouth becomes dry. You have difficulty swallowing, feel as if there is a lump in your throat or as if you might choke. The muscles in your throat feel tight. As you speak, your voice trembles.
- *The heart.* You may notice that your heart has increased its rate of contractions. The pumping of the heart feels quite strong and pounding, as though it could jump out of your chest. It may seem to skip a beat or two. You experience pain or discomfort in your chest.
- *Respiration.* Your rate of breathing increases and becomes more shallow, possibly leading to hyperventilation. You feel as though you cannot take a full, deep breath. You might have difficulty catching your breath, may painfully gasp for air or feel as if you will smother.
- *The stomach.* Your stomach feels full of butterflies or tied in knots. You might feel nauseated.
- *The muscles.* The muscles throughout your body feel tense, especially in the neck and shoulders. If you are driving, you may notice that your hands are gripping the steering wheel so tightly that your knuckles are white and your arms are stiff. In another situation, you may be unconsciously squeezing your hands into fists. Or your muscles may feel weak, your legs unable to keep you standing. Your hands and legs tremble, feel cold, clammy, sweaty, or numb.

In essence, your body, which has been fairly trustworthy over the years, begins to mutiny. And if you experience panic attacks with any frequency, this lack of control slowly erodes your self-confidence and your self-esteem. You begin to restrict your activities to ward off these attacks. Familiar situations become threatening.

- If panic hits you before or during speeches, you begin to turn down speaking engagements.
- If panic shows up while you are traveling, you begin to find excuses for canceling out-of-town business meetings and become "just too busy" to take a vacation with the family.
- If panic intrudes while you are in groups of people, you begin turning down invitations to parties and other gatherings, preferring to stay at home.
- If panic attacks you in stores or restaurants or at the hairdresser's, you begin to avoid any such locations which might stimulate a recurrence of your discomfort.
- If panic appears while you are involved in physical exertion, you begin to avoid any activity that exercises your respiratory or cardiovascular system.
- If panic hits only while you are alone, you begin to cling to your husband or wife, friends, even your children, to ensure safety and protection from this assault by your body.

After you experience several panics, certain doubts creep into your mind: "What is wrong with me? Why is this happening? Am I crazy? Is this the beginning of a nervous breakdown? Are these job [marriage/new baby/house purchase] responsibilities too much for me to handle? Do I have a thyroid condition [heart problem/cancer/high blood pressure]?" For many people, these moments of high excitement or extreme anxiety, of dramatic and sudden changes in the body, are the most frightening and troublesome events of their lives.

It can be difficult to pinpoint the causes of panic; complicating the situation is the fact that anxiety attacks can be found in several psychological disorders and paniclike sensations can be found in dozens of physical disorders. In fact, panic can take place in several contexts. Here are the most common ones.

Panic Within Physical Illness

Some patients with a diagnosed physical problem become susceptible to panic. For instance, patients who have suffered from a heart attack often are cautious of any activity that might place stress on their heart. If they feel their heart increase its pumping action or if they notice a shortness of breath, their worried thoughts can turn to panic: "Oh, no, I've overstressed my heart. Is there any tingling in my arm like before? My chest is beginning to feel tight." Soon, these fearful thoughts can produce such strong sensations that the patient rushes to the hospital emergency room for evaluation. Similar problems arise in those diagnosed with angina, stroke, mitral valve prolapse, asthma, and hypertension.

Such fears during or after a physical illness can have significant repercussions. It has been reported that 95 percent of patients who have had a heart attack begin to suffer from anxiety. Of those discharged from a coronary care unit, 70 percent are given medication to cope with anxiety. In one study of post–heart attack patients who never returned to work, 80 percent remained at home because of psychological causes. Similarly, a study of patients with chronic lung diseases such as emphysema and bronchitis found that 96 percent had disabling anxiety, 74 percent were seriously depressed, and 78 percent were overly preoccupied with their bodies. The fear of becoming breathless seemed to be at the root of most of their problems.

Panic and Dramatic, Frightening Events

Imagine that twice in one week while at the local swimming pool with your young child you watch the lifeguards pull near-drowning children out of the water. You might notice within yourself sensations of anxiety the next time you take your child swimming. This would be a normal response to such an event.

Some people have a more extreme response to that same situation. Their minds become full of horrible fantasies about losing their children. They have strong physical reactions when they consider approaching a pool in the future. This is the type of panic that can arise after a person is involved in any traumatic or frightening event, such as the death of a loved one, a major accident, the diagnosis of a serious illness or an emergency such as a fire or a stuck elevator. When a person reacts with dread or panic in a *harmless* situation and begins to avoid or fear all similar situations, it is defined as a phobia.

Panic, Current Demands and Fearfulness of the Future

Panic may result from fear of the future, regardless of what has actually happened in the past. For many people this occurs when they are faced with increased demands or responsibilities. They may believe that they are incapable of handling the pressures of their responsibilities, that they lack the strength, willpower, skill, intelligence, or emotional stability to cope with some future encounter or task. This fearful anticipation can manifest physically through attacks of extreme anxiety or panic.

Panic and Psychological Disorders

Occasionally, severe anxiety is one part of a more complex psychological disorder. Panic attacks can occur in individuals suffering from problems such as depression, agoraphobia, post-traumatic stress disorder, alcoholism, or obsessive-compulsive disorder.

This book is designed to assist anyone who is suffering from panic attacks, whether they are produced by a fearful response to physical illness, a psychological disorder, some frightening event in the past or future, or the building up of stress from the pressures of daily living.

If you are experiencing some of the physical sensations and psychological reactions described in this chapter, your first obligation is to visit your primary physician for a complete medical examination. Your doctor will identify any physical causes of your problem and will suggest a treatment approach or refer you to a specialist for further evaluation. (Chapter 2 presents the major symptoms of panic that might be caused by physical illness; under each of these symptom categories you will learn about the types of illness involved and any other signs that might indicate a physical problem.)

Once you understand the role—if any—of a physical illness in your discomfort, you can use this book to acquire the understanding and skills necessary to overcome anxiety attacks at the moment they occur. You will learn how the mind may be triggering this emergency reaction in your body. I will describe and illustrate how altering what you think, what you believe, and what you do brings relief from the terror of panic. Your thoughts, beliefs, and actions will play powerful roles as you learn to take control of anxiety attacks.

I will offer relaxation exercises, special breathing patterns, and specific behavioral strategies to use in controlling panic. But change will require more than techniques. You will need to find a new way of looking at old problems. You may discover that your attitudes about life will change as you open your mind to new ideas. And most likely you will learn more about the functions of your body, your mind, and your brain; many of my clients report that they begin to feel relief as soon as they learn that there is a *reason* for these uncomfortable sensations.

There are no simple, universal solutions to life's problems, no magic pills. Any real solution to a complex problem will include a broad and stable foundation from which to build greater strength. You've probably heard the old Chinese proverb: "Give a man a fish and you feed him for a day. Teach a man to fish and you feed him for a lifetime." This book will give you some specific tools to use during the moment of panic. However, to gain control of panic whenever it arises, you must also understand the complex interactions among your body, your mind, your beliefs, and your behavior. In addition, you will find it much easier to conquer these attacks of panic with the support of others, be they professionals, friends, or family.

CHAPTER 2

Physical Causes of
Paniclike Symptoms

E veryone experiences the sensations of anxiety from time
to time. They reflect a normal response to problems arising in our daily lives. In some cases, however, they may
be the signs of a psychological or physical condition. Therein
lies the rub: diagnosing a medical problem is not always a simple
process.

A man complains to his physician that this morning he noticed that his heart was racing, he had difficulty catching his
breath, and he felt dizzy, with tingling around his mouth and in
his hands. He is afraid he is going to die or have a heart attack.
These symptoms could indicate cardiac arrhythmia, pulmonary
embolism, a panic attack, or a hyperventilation episode.

If you are experiencing sensations of panic, there are three
possible diagnoses:

1. A physical disorder is the sole cause of all the sensations associated with panic. Treatment of the physical
   problem removes the discomfort.
2. A minor physical problem is producing a few symptoms.

You become introspective and oversensitive to these sensations and then become anxious. Your heightened awareness and concern produce an increase in discomfort. If this continues, you can turn an insignificant physical problem into major psychological distress.

3. There is no physical basis for the symptoms. That means the problem is psychological and some combination of the following will help: education about the problem, reassurance, self-help skills, psychological treatment, and medication treatment.

This chapter identifies all the major physical problems that can produce paniclike symptoms. By no means should you use this chapter (or any other in this book) for self-diagnosis. Only a physician has the resources to determine whether a physical disorder is the cause of your discomfort and to advise you of your treatment options. In most cases, curing the physical illness or adjusting medication will eliminate the symptoms. In some disorders the symptoms remain as part of a minor disturbance and you must learn to cope with them.

When a person suffers from anxiety attacks, one of the greatest obstacles to recovery can be the fear that these attacks are the indication of a major physical illness—and in rare cases that is true. But most often, when a person continually worries about physical illness, that kind of worry intensifies or even *produces* panic attacks. In other words, the less you worry, the healthier you will become. For that reason, I strongly recommend that you adopt the following guidelines if you are experiencing anxiety attacks:

1. Find a physician whom you *trust*.
2. Explain your symptoms and your worries to that physician.
3. Let your physician conduct any evaluations or ex-

aminations necessary to determine the cause of your symptoms.

4. If your primary physician recommends that another medical specialist evaluate your problem, be certain to follow that advice. Make sure that your primary physician receives a report from the specialist.

5. If a physical problem is diagnosed, follow your physician's treatment advice.

6. If your doctor finds no physical cause for your anxiety attacks, use the methods presented in this book to take control of your reaction to your discomfort. If the problem persists, ask your physician or some other source for a referral to a licensed mental health professional who specializes in treating anxiety disorders (see Chapter 3). You can also email me and I'll do the best I can to refer you to a specialist near you.

The most destructive thing you can do when faced with panic attacks is to steadfastly believe that your physical discomfort means that you have a serious physical illness, despite continued professional reassurance to the contrary. That is why it is essential that you work with a physician whom you can trust until he or she reaches a diagnosis. No matter how many consultations with other professionals you need, allow only *one* professional to take primary charge of your case and receive all reports. Do not continually jump from doctor to doctor. If you remain fearfully convinced that you have a physical ailment, even when there is a consensus to the contrary among the professionals who have evaluated you, then you can be certain of one thing: your fear is directly contributing to your panic episodes. In Parts III and IV you will learn how to control that fear and thereby take control of your anxiety.

Many physical disorders produce paniclike symptoms. Let's look at the symptoms themselves and their possible sources.

Physiological Disorders with Paniclike Symptoms

Cardiovascular Disorders

Angina pectoris
Arrhythmia
Coronary artery disease
Heart attack
Heart failure
Hypertension
Mitral valve prolapse
Mitral stenosis

Myocardial infarction (recovery from)
Postural orthostatic hypotension
Pulmonary edema
Pulmonary embolism
Stroke
Tachycardia
Transient ischemic attack

Respiratory Disorders

Asthma
Bronchitis
Collagen disease

Emphysema
Hypoxia
Pulmonary fibrosis

Endocrine/Hormonal Disorders

Carcinoid tumor
Hyperthyroidism
Hypoglycemia

Pheochromocytoma
Premenstrual syndrome
Pregnancy

Neurological/Muscular Disorders

Compression neuropathies
Guillain-Barré syndrome

Myasthenia gravis
Temporal lobe epilepsy

Ear Disorders

Benign positional vertigo
Labyrinthitis
Mastoiditis

Ménière's disease
Otitis media

Hematic (Kidney) Disorders

Anemia
B_{12} anemia
Folic acid anemia

Iron-deficiency anemia
Sickle cell anemia

(continued on next page)

Physiological Disorders with Paniclike Symptoms *(continued)*

Drug-related Disorders

Alcohol use or withdrawal
Illicit drug use
Medication withdrawal

Side effects of many medications
Stimulant use

Miscellaneous Disorders

Caffeinism
Head injury

Rapid or Irregular Heart Rate

Uncomfortable changes in heart rate are the most frequently reported symptoms of panic attacks. More than 80 percent of those experiencing panic cite a rapid or irregular heart rate as a symptom.

Three complaints are common among patients who seek a doctor's advice about their heart: "My heart feels like it's pounding violently in my chest," "My heart is racing," and "My heart feels like it skips a beat." An arrhythmia is any irregularity in the heart's rhythm. If the heart beats more rapidly than normal, this arrhythmia is called tachycardia. The awareness of an unpleasant sensation in the heart, whether rapid or slow, regular or irregular, is called a palpitation. Heart palpitation is typically an expected sensation when the force and rate of the heartbeat are considerably elevated. After strenuous exercise we are apt to notice the thumping of our heart against the chest wall. As we be-

---

Physical Causes of Rapid or Irregular Heart Rate

Arrhythmia
Tachycardia

Post–myocardial infarction
Organic heart disease

(continued on next page)

Physical Causes of Rapid or Irregular Heart Rate (*continued*)

Palpitation	Heart failure
Extrasystole	Infections
Coronary artery disease	

---

gin resting, that sensation may continue briefly until we recover from our exertion.

People prone to anxiety may have palpitations more frequently when they find themselves in psychologically uncomfortable situations. In fact, the great majority of complaints about the heart presented to physicians indicate a psychological rather than a physical problem. Anxious people may turn their attention to their physical discomfort instead of learning to cope with the situation causing the trouble. After several episodes in which they experience their heart "pounding" or "beating too fast," they fear it is a sign of heart disease or some other physical disorder.

It is possible consciously to notice a few minor disturbances of the heart rhythm. For instance, some people describe sensations such as a "flop" of the heart, the heart "skipping a beat" or "turning a somersault." We call this sudden forceful beat followed by a longer than usual pause an extrasystole. These premature contractions are usually of no serious significance; in fact, arrhythmias of all kinds are common in normal, healthy individuals. In a study published in the *New England Journal of Medicine,* Dr. Harold Kennedy found that healthy subjects with frequent and complex irregular heartbeats seem to be at no more risk of physical problems than is the normal population. In general, researchers are finding that the majority of even the healthiest people have rhythm disturbances such as skipped beats, palpitations, or pounding in the chest.

Tachycardia, or rapid heartbeat, is the most common complaint associated with the heart and is one typical reason that patients seek medical attention. For many normal, healthy individuals it is a daily occurrence in response to physical exercise or intense emotion. Any kind of excitement or trauma, even fatigue or exhaustion, can accelerate the action of the heart, especially in overly anxious individuals. Too many cigarettes, too much alcohol, and in particular, excessive amounts of caffeine can cause tachycardia on occasion. Infections such as pneumonia, as well as acute inflammatory diseases such as rheumatic fever, may also produce a rapid heartbeat.

Although most complaints of palpitations reflect a minor cardiac problem or a sign of anxiety, it is possible that they involve some kind of coronary artery disease. A narrowing of the arteries to the heart causes such diseases. (See also "Chest Pain" below.)

Recovery and rehabilitation after a heart attack can be a difficult psychological challenge. Many people become afraid that too much activity or excitement might produce a second attack. It is no wonder, then, that post–myocardial infarction patients become fearfully preoccupied with the sensations of their heart. Many will return to their doctor's office or hospital emergency room with complaints of palpitations. Fourteen percent of cardiac patients later suffer from panic disorder, which is the worried anticipation of having an anxiety attack or heart attack (discussed in more detail in Chapter 3). Chapter 6 describes the way in which panic complicates recovery from a myocardial infarction.

Complaints of a racing heart can signal certain kinds of organic heart disease and heart failure. More often, however, the symptom of these ailments will be breathlessness. (See also "Difficulty Breathing" below.) Infections such as pneumonia and rheumatic fever may also produce a rapid heartbeat.

Chest Pain

Almost 40 percent of people with panic attacks experience chest pain. The thought that this pain might be a serious heart problem—even though it isn't—sends many sufferers to the emergency room for help. In fact, about 25 percent of patients with chest pain who come to a hospital emergency room (ER) have panic disorder, not any kind of physical problem. The unfortunate news is that of all those panic disorder patients who enter the ER with complaints of chest pain, *98 percent of the time* the ER physicians fail to diagnose panic disorder. Only 15 percent of panic patients who visit their family doctor with chest pain get the proper diagnosis.

The predominant complaint of those suffering from coronary artery disease is most likely to be a pain or pressure in the center of the chest. They may also feel similar discomfort elsewhere in the chest or in the neck, jaw or left arm and occasionally may notice tachycardia (rapid heartbeat).

Angina pectoris is an acute pain in the chest caused by interference with the supply of oxygen to the heart. It is a distinct pain, usually concentrated on the left side and sometimes spreading ("radiating") to the neck and down the left arm. The feeling is of tightness, strangling, heaviness or suffocation. It is not a disease, but a symptom of some underlying disorder that reduces the supply of oxygen to the heart. Coronary artery disease or hypertension are the most common causes, with aortic stenosis, anemia, or hyperthyroidism also possible causes.

Physical Causes of Chest Pain

Coronary artery disease
Angina pectoris
Heart attack

A heart attack (myocardial infarction, coronary thrombosis) occurs when the blood supply to the heart is significantly blocked. The main symptom is usually a crushing pain in the center of the chest, which may continue into the neck, jaw, arms, and stomach. The pain may begin during exercise or a stressful event. Unlike angina, this pain does not stop when the exercise or event ends. A heart attack is a medical emergency. Medical help is needed immediately.

Difficulty Breathing

Dyspnea is difficult, labored, or uncomfortable breathing and can be a signal of a serious emergency or of a mysterious medical puzzle. Seek immediate professional evaluation if this problem has never been diagnosed. Most often a person will describe it as "not being able to catch my breath," or "not getting enough air," while appearing to breathe normally. Certainly the inability to breathe properly can be alarming, and many persons will immediately react with anxiety, fear, or panic.

Physical Causes of Dyspnea (Difficult Breathing)

Bronchitis	Pneumothorax
Emphysema	Hemothorax
Asthma	Pulmonary edema
Pneumoconiosis	Mitral stenosis
Collagen disease	Left ventricular failure
Pulmonary fibrosis	Aortic insufficiency
Myasthenia gravis	Pericardial effusion
Guillain-Barré syndrome	Cardiac arrhythmia
Pleural effusion	

Under normal circumstances, difficult breathing comes after any strenuous activity. If the degree of the problem seems out of proportion to the amount of exertion, concern is appropriate. Troubled breathing is sometimes experienced in pregnancy, since the uterus expands upward, reducing the possibility of a full inhalation. Severe obesity can also reduce the capacity of the lungs to inhale fully.

Most physical causes of dyspnea are associated with disorders of the respiratory and cardiac systems. Acute and chronic diseases of the lungs are the most common physical causes. Within the respiratory system, the problem usually stems from an obstruction of air flow (obstructive disorders) or the inability of the chest wall or lungs to expand freely (restrictive disorders). Each disorder makes the patient work harder to take each breath and decreases the amount of oxygen absorbed with inhalation. The three major obstructive disorders are bronchitis, emphysema, and asthma. In these problems a second common symptom is "chest tightness" upon awakening, shortly after sitting up, or after physical exertion.

The primary symptom of bronchitis is a deep cough that brings up yellowish or grayish phlegm from the lungs. With emphysema, the shortness of breath gradually worsens over the years. The distinct symptoms of bronchitis and the gradual onset of emphysema will usually prevent these disorders from being misdiagnosed as severe anxiety or panic.

Those suffering from asthma complain of difficulty breathing, a painless tightness in the chest and periodic attacks of wheezing. Severe cases can cause sweating, increased pulse rate and severe anxiety. The primary trigger of an asthma attack is an allergy to things such as pollen, dust, or the dander of cats or dogs. Attacks can also be caused by infections, exercise, or psychological stress or may occur for no apparent reason. Some asthma sufferers anxiously anticipate the next attack, since an acute attack of asthma can come suddenly and last for an uncomfortably long time. This fear of an impending attack can actually increase the likelihood of the attack and can extend the length of each attack. Asthma is a good example of a physical disorder that can increase in severity because of anxiety or panic. Chapter 6 describes the way panic can contribute to difficulties in patients with chronic obstructive pulmonary disease (COPD). Special attention is given to chronic bronchitis, emphysema, and asthma.

A number of restrictive disorders of the respiratory system cause difficult breathing. Some produce a rigidity of the lungs (pneumoconiosis, collagen disease, pulmonary fibrosis); others involve the interactions of muscles and nerves (myasthenia gravis, Guillain-Barré syndrome); and still others prevent the lungs from expanding to full volume (pleural effusion, pneumothorax, hemothorax). A restrictive deficit in pulmonary function can also be caused by pulmonary edema, which usually stems from heart failure or occasionally from toxic inhalants.

Dyspnea may occur in any of the various diseases of the heart and lungs, but it is more prominent in those associated with lung congestion. For example, mitral stenosis occurs when a small valve between the left upper and left lower chambers of the heart (the left atrium and left ventricle) becomes abnormally narrow. As blood is forced through the heart, pressure backs up into the lungs and produces congestion, causing breathlessness.

Other possible cardiovascular problems that can lead to difficulty breathing include left ventricular failure, aortic insufficiency, pericardial effusion, and cardiac arrhythmia.

Dizziness and Vertigo

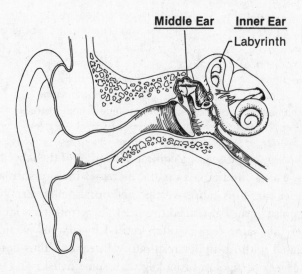

Figure 1. Cross-section of the ear.

The terms *dizziness* and *vertigo* cover a broad range of complaints. Dizziness is a broad term that can include light-headedness, faintness, wooziness, a "swimming" sensation in the head, a floating feeling, double vision, and a feeling of "everything spinning in circles" or of whirling in space. Vertigo refers to the more specific sensations that either the body or its surroundings are turning or the head is swaying or revolving. The physical causes of these two symptoms are numerous, including problems of the middle and inner ear, dental problems, infections, head injuries, drug effects, and disorders of the cardiovascular, neurologic, and central nervous systems.

The ear is responsible for our sense of balance as well as our hearing. The inner ear includes a structure called the labyrinth, which monitors the brain. When injury or infection disrupts the action of the labyrinth, vertigo may occur.

Physical Causes of Dizziness and Vertigo

Ménière's disease	Hypertension
Labyrinthitis	Postural orthostatic hypotension
Nystagmus	Stroke
Benign positional vertigo	Cerebral thrombosis
Ear infections	Cerebral embolism
Dental problems	Cerebral hemorrhage
Head injuries	Transient ischemic attack

In Ménière's disease, a common disorder of the labyrinth in adults, excess fluid builds up and increases the pressure within the inner ear. This causes vertigo and occasionally a ringing or other noise in the ear (called tinnitus). Labyrinthitis is an infection of this same region, often caused by a virus, sometimes associated with an upper-respiratory infection. This can produce severe vertigo, occasionally with some nausea and vomiting during the first episode. The individual may also experience a rapid flickering of the eyes (called nystagmus). Calcium crys-tals floating within the labyrinth can cause benign positional vertigo. In this condition, a shifting of position, such as rolling over in bed, can produce vertigo and nystagmus moments later, lasting no more than thirty seconds. Several kinds of ear infec-tion, such as otitis media and mastoiditis, can cause vertigo, but they also have other distinguishing symptoms, such as drainage of fluid, fever, or redness of the eardrum. Because the teeth and jaw are so closely aligned with the ear, dental problems such as an abscessed tooth, malocclusion, or temporomandibular joint (TMJ) abnormalities can also produce vertigo.

Any head injury can cause a cerebral or labyrinthine concus-sion, which may result in vertigo or a sense of feeling dazed, unsteady, or faint.

A number of cardiovascular and neurovascular diseases may affect a person's sense of balance. Hypertension, or high blood pressure, is often a symptomless disease. However, a swimming or woozy sensation may be the initial symptom that brings a patient into a physician's office for evaluation.

If you experience dizziness and light-headedness when you rise in the morning or change from a lying to an upright posi-tion, postural orthostatic hypotension may be the cause. This is a problem of hypotension, or low blood pressure, and results in poor circulation of blood through the body. Typically, when a person shifts position, the blood vessels reflexively contract to maintain proper blood pressure. In hypotension, this mecha-nism fails to respond appropriately. Since the needed pressure is not maintained, the flow of blood to the brain is temporarily re-duced, causing dizziness and even fainting. Diabetes, minor complications in pregnancy, or hardening of the arteries can cause postural hypotension. It can also be a side effect of antide-pressant medication, major tranquilizers, and even medications prescribed for high blood pressure (hypertension).

The most serious vascular ailment, one that requires imme-diate medical attention, is stroke. When the blood supply to the brain is significantly altered, a stroke occurs and causes damage to the brain. Three types of vascular problems produce stroke: cerebral thrombosis, cerebral embolism, and cerebral hemorrhage. In cerebral thrombosis, some portion of an artery that supplies blood to the brain has been reduced in size. A large deposit of fatty tissue in that portion allows blood to clot, causing a partial or complete blockage of the blood flow to the brain. A cerebral embolism occurs when a bit of blood clot or arteriosclerotic plaque from the heart or the wall of a large artery breaks off and travels to an artery within the brain, where it lodges and causes the stroke. In a cerebral hemorrhage, the artery leaks or bursts, causing blood to seep into the surrounding brain tissues.

A transient ischemic attack is usually caused by a small blood clot or piece of fatty tissue. While passing through the brain, it briefly becomes lodged in a blood vessel, reducing the blood flow through that area. These symptoms resemble those of stroke, but are temporary and do not cause serious harm, since the clot or embolus eventually is dislodged. Although emergency medical attention is not necessary, a transient ischemic attack does require medical evaluation and possible measures to prevent a recurrence.

Dizziness alone is insufficient cause to fear stroke. However, if you experience one or more of the following symptoms, you should consult your physician: numbness and/or tingling in any part of the body, blurred vision, confusion, difficulty speaking, or loss of movement in the arms or legs. These symptoms can also indicate a panic attack rather than stroke. If you experienced such a reaction several times and your doctor finds no sign of a physical disorder, you should consider the possibility that the symptoms are expressions of some psychological, not physical, disturbance.

Multiple Symptoms

Many physical illnesses can produce nervousness in individuals who are not emotionally troubled. Certain other physical disorders—those discussed in this section—can cause a cluster of symptoms that resemble those of panic.

Hypertension is the predominant cardiovascular disorder that can produce multiple symptoms. It is caused by a narrowing of the arteries. As your heart pumps blood through your body it exerts pressure on the arterial walls. If these passageways become constricted, it requires greater force to maintain a steady flow of blood. The entire circulatory system is then under strain, and hypertension is the diagnosis. As mentioned earlier, this is often a symptomless disease, but you might notice symptoms such as palpitations, nervousness, dizziness, and fatigue, as well as a general sense of ill health.

Physical Causes of Multiple Symptoms

Hypertension	Carcinoid syndrome
Mitral valve prolapse	Compression neuropathies
Menopause	Temporal lobe epilepsy
Premenstrual syndrome	Caffeinism
Hyperthyroidism	Amphetamines
Hypoglycemia	Cocaine
Pheochromocytoma	Phencyclidine (PCP)
Anemia	Hallucinogens
Iron deficiency anemia	Marijuana
Folic acid anemia	Alcohol withdrawal
B_{12} anemia	Pulmonary embolism
Sickle-cell anemia	Withdrawal from antidepressants,
Heart attack	narcotics, sedatives,
Hypoxia	barbiturates, benzodiazepines,
	or beta-blockers

Mitral valve prolapse is a condition found in approximately 5 to 15 percent of the adult population. In this disturbance a valve leaflet within the heart balloons into the left upper chamber—the left atrium—of the heart during contraction. About half of all people with mitral valve prolapse complain of heart palpitation sometime in their lives. Other possible symptoms are rapid heartbeat, shortness of breath, dizziness, and an increased awareness of the heart's action (palpitations). This is a rather minor cardiac problem, but people can mistakenly pinpoint it as the sole cause of panic attacks. More often, though, it is the patient's fearful preoccupation with the action of his heart that produces panic. You'll learn more about mitral valve prolapse in Chapter 6.

There is growing evidence that hormonal changes can dramatically affect a person's physical disposition and mood. Approximately 50 percent of women experiencing menopause report some major physical and/or emotional changes. Another 25 percent have uncomfortable, even distressing, symptoms that can include intense moments of palpitations, sweating, hot flashes, and anxiety. Premenstrual syndrome (PMS) refers to a complex of symptoms, including panic, occurring the days just before menstruation. You will learn more about premenstrual syndrome in Chapter 5.

Hyperthyroidism is the overactivity of the thyroid gland and another hormone-caused problem. The thyroid gland is located in the lower front part of the neck and is controlled by a thyroid-stimulating hormone produced in the pituitary gland. In hyperthyroidism, the normal control mechanisms are disrupted and the thyroid continues to produce an excessive amount of its own hormone, thyroxine. This overproduction causes a general speeding up of all chemical reactions in the body. The person may feel shaky and anxious, with heart palpitations, breathlessness, and increased perspiration—as though experiencing a constant anxiety attack. Additional symptoms make this disorder easier to diagnose: thinning hair, chronic tension, increased appetite associated with weight loss instead of gain, and a sense of needing to keep moving despite fatigue and physical exhaustion. Instead of feeling cold, as the anxious person might, the person suffering from hyperthyroidism will feel hot and the skin will be warm to the touch. Your doctor may order a thyroid screening test for you if you have several of these symptoms. Physicians treat hyperthyroidism in one of three ways: through antithyroid medication, by surgically removing either a lump in the thyroid or the whole thyroid, or more commonly, by administering a radioactive iodine fluid that controls the overactivity of the gland.

Hypoglycemia produces several unpleasant symptoms caused by a lower than normal level of glucose in the bloodstream. This state of low blood sugar generally produces a feeling of being uncomfortable, with cold, clammy skin and profuse sweating. Other symptoms can be dizziness, weakness, trembling, tingling in the lips and hands, palpitations, and fainting. The condition is most often found in people with diabetes who take insulin. Many people without diabetes mistakenly believe that hypoglycemia is the cause of their panic symptoms and therefore fail to explore other possible diagnoses. For further information on hypoglycemia and panic, see Chapter 5.

The adrenal glands are located on top of each kidney. The adrenal medulla produces two hormones that play an important role in controlling your heart rate and blood pressure: epinephrine (adrenaline) and nonepinephrine (nonadrenaline). Very rarely a growth, or tumor, develops within or near an adrenal gland and causes an increase in the production of these hormones. Tachycardia, sweating, anxiety, faintness, nausea, and pallor—all resembling sensations of panic—can occur as a result of slight exercise, exposure to cold temperatures, or minor emotional upset. Typically the blood pressure becomes extremely high and the patient may have the frightening feeling of being about to die. This extremely rare disorder, called pheochromocytoma, is cured by surgically removing the tumor.

Anemia is the abnormal decrease of either hemoglobin or red blood cells. Red blood cells carry oxygen from the lungs to all parts of the body. Within each red blood cell is the protein hemoglobin, which combines with the oxygen while in the lungs and then releases it into the tissues as the blood circulates through the body. Characteristic symptoms of anemia are light-headedness, rapid heartbeat, difficulty breathing, and faintness. The anemic person may experience palpitations because the heart is attempting to compensate for the lower levels of oxygen by pumping blood faster than normal. A diagnosis of iron deficiency anemia means that lower than normal levels of iron in the body are limiting the production of hemoglobin. Folic acid anemia and B_{12} anemia mean that the body has insufficient amounts of these two essential vitamins, which are required for the production of healthy red blood cells. Sickle cell anemia is an inherited disease found almost exclusively among people of African descent. In this condition, the red blood cells contain an abnormal hemoglobin, called hemoglobin S. It is associated with a deformed, sickle-shaped cell, which impedes the smooth flow of blood into smaller vessels. Premature destruction of red blood cells, and anemia, result. A physician should diagnose and treat all forms of anemia.

Pulmonary embolism occurs when a blood clot detaches from the wall of a deep vein, moves through the bloodstream and becomes lodged in the pulmonary artery close to or within the lungs. This reduces the volume of fresh blood returning to the left side of the heart and may produce sudden chest pain, rapid heart rate (tachycardia), rapid shallow breathing, and coughing up of bright red spit.

Hypoxia is the diminished availability of oxygen to the body tissues. It is a symptom of several possible underlying problems such as altitude sickness or a pulmonary disorder. Symptoms can include difficulty breathing (dyspnea), rapid pulse, fainting, and chest pain (angina pectoris).

A carcinoid tumor is a small yellow growth occurring in the small intestine, appendix, stomach, or colon. Carcinoid syndrome develops when a carcinoid tumor produces excess amounts of serotonin, a blood vessel constrictor. Exertion, intense emotion, or food or alcohol intake can trigger one or more of the following symptoms: brief flushing of the neck and face, brief abdominal pain, diarrhea, racing heart (tachycardia), low blood pressure (hypotension), facial puffiness, and difficulty breathing caused by bronchoconstriction. Carcinoid tumors are rare.

Compression neuropathies, such as carpal tunnel syndrome, are disorders caused by some form of compression to localized nerves. Symptoms may include a tingling or "pins and needles" feeling similar to symptoms that occur during hyperventilation.

The symptoms of a temporal lobe epilepsy (TLE) attack are highly variable, but in some cases sufferers experience them only as a sudden attack of immense fear or panic. In 60 percent of the cases, fear is the primary emotion. The patient may also have a feeling of unreality, as though he is far away from his surroundings (derealization) or may feel that his body is strange or dreamlike (depersonalization). Highly charged emotional responses can lead to a misdiagnosis of the problem as a psychologically based one. A distinguishing feature of a TLE attack can be the victim's sensing an aura, a sudden experience that often takes the form of a strange aroma or taste at the moment of fear.

Caffeinism refers to the uncomfortable side effects that can occur with high intake of caffeine from coffee, tea, cola drinks, chocolate, and over-the-counter medication such as Excedrin and Anacin. Symptoms include anxiety, irritability, insomnia, headaches, stomach irritation, agitation, increased respiration, rapid heartbeat, and irregular heart rhythm. These side effects can occur with daily consumption of 250 to 500 mg. Between 20 and 30 percent of Americans consume more than 500 mg of caffeine a day (equal to four to five cups of drip coffee). Some panic-prone persons are highly sensitive to caffeine, and symptoms can occur from less caffeine intake than the average person. If you experience any of these symptoms, you may wish to review your intake of all forms of caffeine. Use the following tables as a guide.

Presence of Caffeine

Medications (per tablet/capsule)

Vivarin	200 mg	Fiorinal	40 mg
Dextrin	200 mg	Medigesic	40 mg
Cafergot	100 mg	Empirin	32 mg
No Doz	100 mg	Esgic	40 mg
Excedrin	65 mg	Midol	32 mg
Fiorecet	40 mg	Anacin	32 mg

Coffees, Teas, and Cocoa (per 5–6 oz serving, except where noted) / Cola Beverages (per 12 oz can)

Starbucks (16 oz)	372 mg	Coke	64 mg
Starbucks (12 oz)	279 mg	Diet Coke	45 mg
Drip coffee	115–175 mg	Dr. Pepper (reg. & diet)	41 mg
Drip coffee, automatic	137 mg	Mellow Yellow	51 mg
Instant coffee	60 mg	Mountain Dew (reg. & diet)	55 mg
Decaffeinated coffee	3 mg	Mr. Pibb	40 mg
Green tea	35 mg	Pepsi Cola, Diet Pepsi	38 mg
Black tea	70 mg	7-Up, Sprite, Fresca, Hire's Root Beer	0 mg
Instant tea	33 mg		
Decaffeinated tea	1 mg		
Hot cocoa	5–13 mg		

Energy Drinks

Redline RTD	250 mg	XS	83 mg
Monster	160 mg	Red Bull	80 mg
Full Throttle	144 mg	Amp	83 mg

Chocolate

Baking chocolate (1 oz)	25 mg	Milk chocolate (1 oz)	1–15 mg
Dark chocolate (1 oz)	5–35 mg	Chocolate milk (8 oz)	5 mg

Amphetamines, whether taken for treatment of depression, for weight control, or illicitly for recreation, can cause severe anxiety to the point of panic. This extreme reaction is also possible with illicit drugs such as cocaine and phencyclidine (PCP) and the hallucinogens such as LSD and mescaline. Marijuana causes increased heart rate that can lead to a severe anxiety reaction.

Alcohol withdrawal can produce nervousness, rapid heartbeat, confusion, high blood pressure and panic, as well as other symptoms. Too rapid withdrawal, especially after long-term use, from antidepressants, narcotics, sedatives, barbiturates, benzodiazepines, or beta-blockers can cause symptoms such as anxiety, rapid heartbeat, high blood pressure, and panic.

Side Effects of Medications

Sometimes a medication may cause unwanted side effects along with its needed effects. If these occur, you should check with your doctor. In addition to other possible side effects, each of the medications listed below may produce paniclike symptoms. All medications are listed by their generic names.

- *Aminophylline* relieves shortness of breath and wheezing in acute bronchial asthma and is prescribed to reduce asthmalike symptoms in chronic bronchitis and emphysema. Side effects can include nervousness, rapid heartbeat, and dizziness.
- *Antidepressants* are used to treat depression and panic attacks. (See Chapter 20 regarding the use of antidepressants within the treatment of panic.) Possible side effects are increased anxiety or agitation, dizziness, and irregular or rapid heartbeat.
- *Antidyskinetics* are used in the treatment of Parkinson's disease. Side effects may include dizziness, irregular heartbeat, and anxiety.
- *Atropine* is a medication used to dilate the pupil of the

eye. It can produce an unusually fast heartbeat. A number of drugs are atropinelike in their effects. These are usually called anticholinergic medications.

- *Isoproterenol and metaproterenol (Alupent)* are inhaler forms of beta-Z adrenergic agents that relieve acute bronchial asthma and bronchospasms associated with chronic bronchitis and emphysema. Side effects can include general anxiety, dizziness, rapid and strong heartbeat, and shaky hands.

- *Cycloserine* is an antibiotic medication whose side effects may include anxiety, irritability, confusion, dizziness, and restlessness.

- *Digitalis* is prescribed to improve the strength and efficiency of the heart or to control the rate of the heartbeat. It can produce an unusually slow or uneven pulse.

- *Ephedrine* is prescribed for lung problems. Side effects can be nervousness, restlessness, dizziness, difficulty breathing, palpitations, and rapid heartbeat.

- *Epinephrine* is used in the treatment of the eyes, the lungs, and allergies. Side effects can include faintness, trembling, rapid heartbeat, palpitations, nervousness, and difficulty breathing.

- *Insulin* helps control diabetes. Increasing the dose of insulin can occasionally trigger a hypoglycemic reaction, which includes sweating, cold clammy hands, dizziness, palpitations, and trembling.

- *Isoniazid,* an anti-infection medication, may produce rapid heartbeat and light-headedness.

- *Monoamine oxidase inhibitors (MAOIs)* are in the antidepressant family. Physicians prescribe them to reduce symptoms of depression and also to treat panic attacks (see Chapter 20). Possible side effects are dizziness or light-headedness—especially when getting up from a lying or sitting position—and rapid or pounding heartbeat.

- *Nitrates* are used to improve the blood flow to the heart and to relieve angina. Possible side effects are dizziness, light-headedness, and rapid heartbeat.
- *Prednisone* is the most commonly used of the corticosteroids and is prescribed to relieve inflammation. Its side effects can include irregular heartbeat, nervousness, muscle weakness, and mood swings. Other corticosteroid medications may cause similar side effects.
- *Reserpine* is used to treat high blood pressure and certain emotional conditions, as well as a few other problems. Side effects may include dizziness, faintness, anxiety, and palpitations. Some individuals can develop phobic reactions while taking reserpine.
- *Synthetic thyroid hormones* are used for treating hypothyroidism. Excessive levels of these hormones can cause rapid heartbeat, palpitations, shortness of breath, nervousness, unusual sweating, and anxiety.

CHAPTER 3

Panic within
Psychological Disorders

I f your panic is persisting, you have probably become increasingly alarmed. Even when you can identify what you believe to be the immediate cause of these intense moments of anxiety, you are left with a bewildering array of questions: "Why me? Why now? What does it mean? How serious is it? How do I stop it?"

Few panic sensations continue because of a physical problem. Most difficulties, even if associated with a physical disorder, are sustained through a psychological response to the experience. For instance, cardiac patients have suffered a physical trauma associated with the heart. One study found that up to 14 percent of these patients can also be diagnosed with panic disorder. Their episodes of severe anxiety start after their heart problems but are not caused by it. If the physical trauma were the cause, then more people who have heart problems would also suffer from panic attacks. The anxiety stems from the way cardiac patients react to the event. The more fearful they become about the prospect of another physical trauma to the heart, the greater their chances of suffering from extreme anxiety or panic.

Not everyone is so troubled by anxiety that they suffer from a psychological disorder. Some people simply pass through a difficult time—job changes or family conflicts—with some level of anxiety, then continue on their way. However, if the troubles remain over time, they will usually fall within one of seven different categories of psychological problems: panic disorder, agoraphobia, generalized anxiety disorder, phobias, social anxiety disorder, obsessive-compulsive disorder, and post–traumatic stress disorder.

Panic Disorder

Panic disorder is the only psychological problem whose predominant feature is recurring panic (or anxiety) attacks. Although the first panic attack may take place in a distinct situation, later episodes may be unpredictable as to time or place. After a number of panic episodes, it's common to become afraid of being a helpless victim of panic. You may hesitate to be alone, to venture far from home or to be in public places. Even when not experiencing an anxiety attack, the person with panic disorder often becomes increasingly nervous and apprehensive and remains physically and psychologically tense in preparation for the next attack.

The physical sensations are the same as those described in Chapter 1. One or more of these can be present in a severe form during an actual panic attack or in a milder form at other times: dry mouth; sweating; acute tension in the stomach, back of neck, or shoulders; increased heart rate; dizziness or light-headedness; feeling faint; increased respiration; trembling hands, legs, or voice; weak, numb, or cold extremities; shortness of breath; body fatigue; difficulty swallowing; a lump in the throat; irritability; blurred vision; inability to concentrate; and confusion.

The first panic attack may seem to appear without warning, yet it typically comes during an extended period of stress. This stress is not caused by a few days of tension, but extends over several months. Life transitions such as moving, job change, marriage, or the birth of a child often account for much of the psychological pressure.

For some individuals, learning to manage this stressful period, or to reduce the pressures, will eliminate the panic episodes. For others, it is as though the stress of the life transition or problem situation uncovered a psychological vulnerability. If the panic-prone accept increased responsibilities—for instance, a job promotion or the birth of a first child—they may begin to doubt their ability to meet the new demands, the expectation of others, and the increased energy required for these responsibilities. Instead of focusing on mastering the task, they become more concerned with the possibility of failure. This attention to the threat of failure continually undermines their confidence. Through a series of steps, described in Part II of this book, the panic-prone translate these fears into panic.

For some, the uncomfortable sensations will wake them in the middle of the night. These are caused either by panic disorder or are night terrors (known as *pavornocturnus* in children and *incubus* in adults). Most nocturnal panics take place during non-REM sleep, which means they do not tend to come in response to dreams or nightmares. They occur from a half-hour to three-and-a-half hours after the person has fallen asleep and are usually not as severe as daytime panics. These are similar to night terrors since they both produce sudden awakening and autonomic arousal and tend not to be associated with nightmares. However, they are also distinct, since people who experience a night terror tend to have amnesia for it and return to sleep without trouble. They also can become physically active during the terror—tossing, turning, kicking, sometimes screaming loudly or running out of the bedroom in the midst of an episode. Nocturnal panic attacks, however, tend to cause insomnia. The person has a vivid memory of the panic. He does not become physically aggressive during the panic attack, but remains physically aroused after the occurrence and has difficulty going back to sleep.

Panic Disorder with Agoraphobia

The literal meaning of panic disorder with agoraphobia is "fear of the marketplace." Each person who receives the diagnosis can have a unique combination of symptoms. But common to all symptoms is a marked fear or avoidance of being alone or in certain public places. It is a response strong enough to significantly limit the individual's normal activities. Although the proper diagnostic term is panic disorder with agoraphobia, to simplify things I'll now refer to it as agoraphobia.

For those experiencing panic attacks, the distinction between agoraphobia and panic disorder is based on how many activities they avoid. Those with panic disorder remain relatively active, although they may avoid a few uncomfortable situations. When they begin to significantly restrict their normal activities because of these fearful thoughts, agoraphobia is the more appropriate diagnosis.

For some people, agoraphobia develops from panic disorder. They become physically and emotionally tense in anticipation of the next attack, so we call this anticipatory anxiety. To reduce the distress, they begin to avoid any circumstances that seem associated with past panic attacks and thus become more and more limited in their range of activities.

The fearful thoughts that plague those with agoraphobia often revolve around *loss of control*. They may fear the development of uncomfortable physical sensations familiar from past experiences, such as dizziness or rapid heartbeat. They may then worry that these could become even worse than they were in the past, such as fainting or having a heart attack. Or they worry that they will become trapped or confined in some physical location or social situation such as a restaurant or party. In the first two situations—fear of fainting or heart attack—they sense that their body is out of control. In the third—feeling trapped—they feel unable to readily control their surroundings. Those with agoraphobia may avoid many of these situations as a way to feel safe. The need to avoid is so strong that some people with agoraphobia will quit their jobs, stop driving, or taking public transportation or stop shopping or eating in restaurants. In the worst cases they never venture outside their home for years.

The following list shows the types of surroundings that can provoke these fears.

Fear of Surroundings

Public Places or Enclosed Spaces

Streets
Stores
Restaurants
Theaters
Churches

Travel

On trains, buses, planes,
  subways, cars
Over bridges, through tunnels
Being far away from home
Traffic

Conflict Situations

Arguments, interpersonal
  conflicts, expression of anger

*Confinement or Restriction of
  Movement*

Barber's, hairdresser's, or
  dentist's chair
Lines at a store
Waiting for appointments
Prolonged conversations in
  person or on phone
Crowds
Remaining at home alone

Open Spaces

Parks
Fields
Wide streets

Listed below are the types of fearful thoughts associated with the dreaded situations. These are irrational, unproductive, and anxiety-producing thoughts that last anywhere from a few seconds to more than an hour. At the same time, these thoughts are the primary cause of agoraphobic behavior; they serve to maintain the belief "If I avoid these situations, I'll be safe."

Fearful Thoughts

Fainting or collapsing in public
Developing severe physical
  symptoms
Losing control
Dying
Causing a scene
Having a heart attack or other
  physical illness

Being trapped or confined
Becoming mentally ill
Being unable to breathe
Becoming confused
Being unable to cope
Being unable to get home or
  to another "safe" place

Some people with agoraphobia will experience no panic. Although fearful thoughts continue to control these individuals, they have restricted their lifestyles, through avoidance, to such a degree that they no longer become uncomfortable.

When those with agoraphobia retreat to protect themselves, they often have to sacrifice friendships, family responsibilities, and careers. Their loss of relationships, affections, and accomplishments compounds the problem. It leads to low self-esteem, isolation, loneliness, and depression. In addition, they may become dependent on alcohol or drugs in an unsuccessful attempt to cope. (See Chapter 4 for further discussion of this complex disorder; see Chapter 5 for the problem of alcoholism. Parts III and IV address the specific ways in which those with agoraphobia can take control of their fears and their anxiety attacks.)

Generalized Anxiety Disorder

With generalized anxiety disorder, panic is not the predominant feature. However, many panic sensations are present to a lesser degree. Instead of brief moments of intense anxiety, the person can feel discomfort throughout most of the day. Although the specific manifestations of anxiety vary for each person, this chronic state of tension can affect six major systems of the body.

1. In the cardiovascular system, anxiety increases blood pressure, which causes tachycardia (rapid heartbeat), constriction of the blood vessels in the arms and legs and dilation of the vessels surrounding the skeletal muscles. These changes produce palpitations (an uncomfortable awareness of the heart rate), headaches, and cold fingers.

2. In the gastrointestinal system, anxiety leads to reduced salivary secretions, spasms within the esophagus (the hollow muscular tube leading from the nose and mouth to the stomach) and alterations in the stomach, intestines, and anal sphincter. These systemic changes result in dry mouth, difficulty swallowing, "butterflies" in the stomach, the gurgling sounds of gas in the intestines, and mucous colitis (an inflammation of the colon), causing spasms, diarrhea, or constipation and cramplike pains in the upper stomach.

3. In the respiratory system, anxiety leads to hyperventilation, or overbreathing, causing "air hunger," deep sighs, and pins-and-needles sensations. This overbreathing lowers the level of carbon dioxide in the blood. (See Chapter 16 for further information on hyperventilation.)

4. In the genitourinary system, the anxious person can experience the need for frequent urination. Men may have difficulty

maintaining an erection during intercourse; women may have difficulty becoming sexually aroused or achieving orgasm.

5. In the musculoskeletal system, the muscles become tense. Involuntary trembling of the body, tension headaches, and other aches and pains may develop.

6. Through changes in the central nervous system, anxious people are generally more apprehensive, aroused, and vigilant, feeling "on edge," impatient, or irritable. They may complain of poor concentration, insomnia, and fatigue.

As you can see, there is often a fine line between the diagnosis of panic disorder and that of generalized anxiety disorder. Three features distinguish them: symptoms, fearful thoughts, and response to fears. When the symptoms cause people to feel chronically anxious (as they can with generalized anxiety disorder) and also experience episodes of panic, then panic disorder or agoraphobia will be the more likely diagnosis.

Different kinds of fearful thoughts are associated with the two problems. In most people with generalized anxiety disorder the worries focus on two or more of these topics: work or school, money, health, and relationships. And over 90 percent of them worry about minor events throughout the day. They will often doubt their abilities in the world: "Will I fail in this work setting?" "Are they going to accept me?" "I'm afraid the kids are going to be harmed." "What if one day I can't pay the mortgage?" "I'll never perform up to their expectations." With panic disorder and agoraphobia, the imagined response of others is secondary to the fear of personal catastrophe or loss of control, and their internal statements and questions will reflect this apprehension: "What if I faint [become hysterical, have a heart attack, cause a scene] and people see me?" The panic-prone focus more on their ability to be in 100 percent control of all their physical and mental capacities. Those with generalized

Possible Physical Sensations During Anxiety

Cardiovascular System

Tachycardia (rapid heartbeat)
Palpitations (uncomfortable
    awareness of the heart rate)

Headaches
Cold fingers

Gastrointestinal System

Dry mouth
Difficulty swallowing
"Butterflies" in the stomach
Gurgling sounds of gas in the
    intestines

Colon spasms
Diarrhea and/or constipation
Cramplike pains in the upper
    stomach

Respiratory System

Hyperventilation (see Chapter 16)

Genitourinary System

Need for frequent urination

Difficulty maintaining an erection
    or feeling arousal

Musculoskeletal System

Muscles tense
Involuntary trembling of the
    body

Tension headaches
Other aches and pains

Central Nervous System

Apprehensive, aroused, and
    vigilant
Feeling "on edge," impatient, or
    irritable
Poor concentration

Insomnia
Fatigue

anxiety focus more on their inability to cope with external events.

People with generalized anxiety respond to fears by thinking about withdrawing from situations that might increase their anxiety and they may procrastinate on performance tasks. People with panic disorder or agoraphobia, on the other hand, are quick to use avoidance as a way to diminish discomfort. In a matter of days they will begin to identify the situations that are associated with their discomfort and determine how they can steer clear of them, immediately viewing avoidance as the single best solution to the problem.

Social Anxiety Disorder

Social anxiety disorder is an excessive, unreasonable fear that others in public will notice and negatively judge some particular activity. People with social anxiety become distressed even at the *thought* of this activity, for fear that they will be humiliated or embarrassed. Avoidance is their primary defense, which they feel compelled to use.

The variety of social anxieties range from those that seem to be an exaggeration of common fears to those that seem bizarre to others. The most prevalent are the fears of speaking or performing in public. Most people understand and have experienced the normal anxiety associated with public speaking: trembling hands and legs, increased perspiration, "butterflies," and worries about performing poorly. Those with social anxiety not only become highly anxious if they are forced to approach such a situation but will do all in their power to avoid it. That's why we sometimes call this social phobia.

Any situation in which others may observe the person's behavior can become a threat: urinating in a public bathroom, signing one's name while being observed, or being watched while eating. One client became anxious in almost every public situation because she feared people would begin watching her eyes.

This belief was so real and so overwhelming that she was in a constant state of anxiety when not in her own home.

Anxiety, potential for panic, and avoidance behavior link social anxiety disorder with panic disorder and agoraphobia. The distinguishing feature is, again, what the person fears. Those with agoraphobia predominantly fear that their body will not perform normally. Those with social anxiety worry about people's reaction to seemingly normal behavior such as eating lunch or walking into a room while others are seated.

People with generalized anxiety can sometimes struggle during a change in their personal life or career life that diminishes their self-confidence. Those with social anxiety, on the other hand, may never have mastered basic social skills. Many report being shy and isolated as children and adolescents, long before this problem began. For these people, social anxiety disorder can be viewed as an extreme manifestation of a long-standing sensitivity to the opinions of others.

Specific Phobias

When a person has a persistent, irrational fear of an object or situation and a strong urge to avoid that object or situation, we call that specific phobia. Most people have met someone with a significant fear of a particular object or situation: closed spaces (claustrophobia), heights (acrophobia), water (aquaphobia), snakes (ophidiphobia), or lightning (astraphobia). The most prevalent phobias are of specific animals and insects, of the natural elements such as storms or water, of heights, and of closed-in spaces.

People with a specific phobia will react with anxiety or even panic when confronted with the prospect of facing the fearful situation. However, their fear is not of their body's sensations (as in panic disorder or agoraphobia) but of the situation itself, which they believe to be dangerous. Some may also fear that they will lose their senses and do something foolish. The person with a height phobia, for instance, might fear that he will forget what he is doing and accidentally leap off the cliff on which he is standing. Others with phobias fear that something will go wrong with their circumstances. The individual with a flying phobia might vividly imagine the tail falling off the plane, or the pilot losing consciousness with no one to take over, or the oxygen in the cabin running out in midflight. Such fears defy rational thinking. Most with phobias know that they are being excessive and unreasonable in their thoughts, but this knowledge is of no use to them. The fearful thoughts come automatically in spite of rational thought and thus the person with a phobia may believe the only recourse is to avoid the problematic area.

Specific phobias may develop rapidly, as after a particular traumatic event, or gradually over the years, sometimes as a result of childhood learning and the examples set by parents and others. For instance, some people didn't gain enough knowledge and experience during their childhood to successfully face new, threatening life experiences—whether real or imaginary—as adults. Instead of gaining some perspective during fearful times, those with a phobia become passive victims of their fear. The only action they take is to back away.

Diagnosing the true fear is an essential part of the cure. For instance, the person with a flying phobia may be afraid of heights or being trapped, being far away from home, having a panic attack, or a combination of these.

When a person has several specific phobias, the relationship between them may not seem evident at first. One agoraphobic patient also developed an intense fear of knives and of children. While discussing the problem during a treatment session, she reported that one day several months earlier she had found her seven-year-old son threatening his sister with a kitchen knife. After admonishing her son, she found herself dwelling on the many dangers of knives. Within a day, she began to question her own ability to control a knife. She then developed a spontaneous mental image of herself hurting a child with a knife. In a brief few days she began avoiding knives as well as becoming anxious whenever she looked at young children. The internal belief that was driving her fear was "I don't have enough self-control [to handle knives, to be with children]." Such a fear is common with those diagnosed with obsessive-compulsive disorder.

Thus, phobias can be more complex than they at first seem. Their "irrational" nature may relate to the person's attempt to solve a real-life problem. After a time the irrational fear response takes on a life of its own, just like a habit. And like a habit, it can be un-learned.

Obsessive-Compulsive Disorder

Obsessive-compulsive disorder (OCD) has two components: obsessions and compulsions. Obsessions are repetitive, anxiety-producing thoughts that almost all of us have experienced from time to time. We can be driving down the road, ten minutes from home, heading for a week's vacation. Suddenly the thought enters our mind, "Did I unplug the iron after I finished with that shirt?" Then we think, "I must have . . . but I don't know, I was rushing around so at the last minute. Did I reach down and pull the cord out of the socket? I can't remember. Was the iron light still on as I walked out the door? No, it was off. Was it? I can't leave it on all week; the house will burn down. This is ridiculous!" Eventually we either turn around and head home to check as the only way to feel relieved, or we convince ourselves that we did indeed take care of the task. This is an example of what can take place inside anyone's mind when we are worrying about a particular problem. In the mind of a person with obsessive-compulsive disorder, this pattern of thought is exaggerated and persistent.

Compulsions are repetitive, unproductive behaviors that people engage in ritualistically. As with obsessive thoughts, most of us have engaged in a few compulsive behaviors sometime in our lives. As children, we played with superstitions, such as never stepping on a sidewalk crack or turning away when a black cat crossed our path. Some of these persist as we become adults— many of us still never walk under a ladder.

OCD, however, is much more serious than these minor habits. Obsessive people are driven by persistent negative thoughts that are involuntary, uncontrollable, and consuming. Self-doubt, ambivalence, indecision, and impulses fill their waking hours. These thoughts and the compulsive actions are a defense against making any mistake. Their internal belief often is "I must do this to prevent anything tragic from happening." At the same time, the person knows that these thoughts are irrational, and he tries to resist them. The more he resists, the stronger they become.

The most common obsessive thoughts are of violence (poisoning one's spouse or stabbing a child), committing an immoral act, doubting whether one has performed some action (turning off the kitchen stove), and contamination (catching germs by picking up objects or touching someone).

Compulsions are also motivated by a need to relieve anxiety through rules or required rituals. Common compulsions are hand washing, sometimes for hours each day, and repetitively checking for safety. One of my clients can illustrate the pattern of many others. She felt compelled to check if she had left the stove on each time she left her house for an errand. She would lock the front door as she was leaving, then feel a strong urge to return to the kitchen and touch each burner control knob as she checked it. As soon as she walked back outside she would doubt herself and again feel a strong urge to repeat the process. After twelve or so times, she usually felt free enough to leave the house. Sometimes, however, this fear forced her to cancel her plans.

High anxiety and even panic can result whenever people attempt to stop the ritual. Tension and anxiety build to such an intense degree that they surrender once again to the thoughts or behaviors. Unlike an alcoholic who feels compelled to drink but also enjoys the drinking experience, people with OCD gain relief through the ritual, but no pleasure.*

Post–Traumatic Stress Disorder

Post–traumatic stress disorder (PTSD) identifies a specific emotional distress that can follow a major psychologically or physically traumatic event. This uncommon event would typically produce fear and anxiety in anyone who experienced it. Examples are rape or assault, a natural disaster, being in or witnessing a serious accident, major surgery, and wartime combat duty. Symptoms may begin immediately or may not surface for six months, a year, or even longer.

Severe anxiety and panic are just two of several possible symptoms. The person will have recurring images of the traumatic event, often with the same degree of anxiety as during the event itself. Or he will suddenly feel as though the event is occurring in the present. Recurring nightmares of the trauma are dramatic and disturbing, and nightmares, anxiety, or depression can disrupt sleep. The person may remain tense and anxious throughout the day and may startle easily.

As they become more physically involved with these experiences, traumatized individuals begin to withdraw from the world, show less emotion, and become uninterested in people and activities that were once important. They avoid any situations that might stimulate memories of the traumatic event. Guilt, depression, and sudden outbursts of aggressive behavior may also surface. Drug and alcohol abuse develop in some as they attempt to manage these responses.

---

* We have written a self-help book specifically for anyone suffering from OCD, titled *Stop Obsessing! How to Overcome Obsessions and Compulsions,* by Dr. Edna Foa and Dr. Reid Wilson. New York: Bantam, 2001.

The largest group to experience this problem are combat veterans. In fact, it was after studies of Vietnam veterans were added to studies of civilian post–trauma sufferers that the American Psychiatric Association created in 1980 the diagnostic category post–traumatic stress disorder. In the United States, the largest percentage of PTSD cases is Vietnam War vets and those returning from combat in the Persian Gulf and Afghanistan. It is speculated by experts that up to one-third of Iraq veterans will develop PTSD.

The major task in overcoming this problem is to help those with PTSD to incorporate the traumatic event into their sense of the world and into their understanding of their personal life. As they get better, they learn to put the trauma into its proper place in the past instead of re-living it as though it is in the present.

CHAPTER 4

Agoraphobia and the
Panic-Prone Personality

The nature of panic disorder with agoraphobia is so complex that it must be viewed as different from all other phobias. It is not the moment of panic that distinguishes agoraphobia, nor is it simply that a broader group of fears is involved. The physiological reactions of someone with claustrophobia who is facing an open elevator can be as severe as those with agoraphobia, and the person with claustrophobia may avoid just as many situations for fear of being trapped. The primary difference between agoraphobia and all other phobias lies in the beliefs that sustain the fear within the individual. These beliefs are often established by the past experiences in life of each person with agoraphobia and can be supported by current relationships as well as memories of the past.

If you experience agoraphobia, you must do more than learn to master the moment of panic. You will need to take every opportunity to learn more about yourself, your relationship with the significant people currently in your life, and your childhood development. The issues in agoraphobia include not only how you feel about frightening situations, but what you think about yourself, how you compare yourself with others, how you treat others, and how you let them treat you.

Learning how to handle your thoughts and your physical sensations as you approach a feared situation is an essential skill, just as it is for people experiencing panic from any source. In addition, though, you must learn about your self-perception and any limitations you feel as a human being. You will need all the strength you can muster to conquer this problem. In this chapter I will show you how self-perception, current relationships, and past relationships or events can set the stage for panic and weaken your stand against fear. In Chapter 3 you read that the major fear within agoraphobia is *loss of control*. Keep that in mind as you read this chapter. I will be illustrating a number of ways that people learn to feel out of control, not only in the panic-provoking situation but in their entire lives.

Studies have found that women constitute about 60 percent of the pure panic disorder cases and 90 percent of panic disorder with agoraphobia. Researchers have not yet determined why this is true. In the years to come we will most likely find that there are many influencing factors. Here are several hypotheses that are not validated by scientific method:

1. Traditionally, parents and our culture have focused little attention on preparing young women to manage independently after leaving their parents' home. Fairy-tale fantasies of the delicate female being protected by the dominant, caring male can be shattered by the actual pressures of marriage, parenthood, and the working world. If young women believe that their skills are no match for the tasks they face, they can become vulnerable to anxiety, self-doubt, and overdependence.

2. Agoraphobia develops more easily within a person who succumbs to the fear of panic by avoiding situations. By continually confronting anxiety, you desensitize yourself to those sensations.

The stereotypical image of the macho male may pressure men to tolerate anxiety and still face fearful situations. In this way, some men learn coping mechanisms that prevent anxieties from building into panic. If women or men allow themselves to give in to fear, they give up ground and agoraphobia steps in.

In this same vein, people who work at home are at a disadvantage compared with those who must travel to work each day to maintain their jobs. Consider a married couple with a new infant, where the husband has a full-time job and the wife is the primary caretaker. If the husband begins to feel panicky as he gets up in the morning, he also feels a strong, competing pressure to tolerate his discomfort and make it to work on time. He feels the responsibility to provide his family with that weekly paycheck; he cannot easily avoid facing work. If the wife begins to feel anxious about going grocery shopping in the morning, her schedule often permits her to postpone the trip until tomorrow. If driving to the park with her child might be anxiety-provoking, they can play at home today. So the spouse with a flexible schedule runs the greater risk of using avoidance to control panic instead of using the more successful methods of direct confrontation. You might say, "She who hesitates is lost." Soon, the need to avoid can become predominant, and agoraphobia develops. This pattern is not gender-based; anyone who has flexibility in their schedule can be more vulnerable to avoidance.

3. Biological differences may play a role in increasing a woman's susceptibility to panic. Changes in the endocrine system are considered the strongest influencing factors. Many women with agoraphobia will have their first struggle with panic after the birth of a child, a time when there are great changes in hormone levels. Others report increased anxiety or increased frequency of panic during their premenstrual week, a time when estrogen and progesterone levels temporarily drop. (Premenstrual syndrome is further discussed in Chapter 5.)

Although these biological factors may prove to be significant in agoraphobia, psychological influences may play an equally important role during postpartum or premenstrual times. Agoraphobia usually develops during a prolonged period of stress. Every mother knows of the surprisingly large number of adjustments she faces physically, psychologically, interpersonally, and economically as a new baby enters her life. Stress stems from the degree of change in one's life, regardless of whether that change is viewed as positive or negative. The stress of new parenthood can take its toll. Regarding premenstrual influences, if a woman regularly experiences physical and emotional discomfort during a certain week each month, then she will inevitably begin to anticipate that week. If she hasn't found any successful way to manage her discomfort, she will most likely anticipate the event with anxiety. In other words, the actual discomfort caused by biological factors is intensified by fearful expectation. This soon leads to a conditioned response: the woman unconsciously begins to brace in preparation for discomfort. Such bracing increases tension levels and makes her more susceptible to panic.

Another biological factor is the difference between the levels of testosterone in males and in females. This hormone, which is found in much higher levels in men, is linked with dominance behavior. Thus men may be somewhat less likely to experience fear and might confront fearful situations more aggressively than women.

4. It is possible that the disproportionate ratio of female to male agoraphobia reflects an underestimation of male agoraphobia. One argument for this hypothesis is the suggestion that men mask their panic sensations through abuse of alcohol (see Chapter 5). That macho male image may stop men from admitting problems or asking for appropriate help, whereas women more readily admit to psychological causes of problems and are more likely to seek out mental-health professionals. Use or abuse of alcohol is a

convenient self-treatment that offers short-term relief. However, when men who struggle with both alcohol and agoraphobia do seek help, they are more likely to end up at Alcoholics Anonymous meetings or alcohol treatment centers than with a mental-health professional who can spot their agoraphobia. A.A. programs directly address the substance-abuse problems but only indirectly offer help with agoraphobia issues.

Since such a small percentage of men have been diagnosed with agoraphobia, our understanding of their difficulties is less developed. As a group, these men seem more extroverted, aggressive, and ambitious than some of the women discussed in this chapter. Their greatest difficulty is in expressing their emotions directly, especially in intimate relationships. For this reason, the first episodes may develop soon after conflicts arise within a marriage. Learning self-confidence within an intimate relationship and learning to accept some of the changing roles of women today may be an important factor in helping some men with agoraphobia.

The Power of Beliefs
Learned in the Past

Each psychological theme in this chapter will be illustrated through the reflections and insights of five women who have suffered from agoraphobia. Before you meet each of them, there are several things you should know. First, these women generously agreed to permit an audio recording of our interviews. All names and biographical information have been altered to protect the confidentiality of our relationship. Second, their childhood experiences are typical of those suffering from severe forms of this disorder. Their long-term struggle with agoraphobia—lasting twelve to fifty years—is common for those who do not receive appropriate professional treatment. With our new treatment approaches designed specifically for agoraphobia, people no longer need to remain trapped by panic for so many years. However, the accounts of these women provide an understanding of the workings of agoraphobia, which could not be so clearly and briefly illustrated by less dramatic cases. Third, it is not within the scope of this book to outline the treatment of all aspects of agoraphobia. Instead, I will describe the women as they appear at the initial stage of treatment and will summarize the therapeutic tasks ahead of them as they learn to control panic attacks. And, fourth, I am limiting the details about their lives to those that help support the themes of this chapter. Many issues come to bear on complex psychophysiological problems, and those issues can be different in each individual.

As each woman shares her story, reflect on whether your experiences or feelings are similar. Take this opportunity to learn about yourself. Each theme that is not a problem for you is a positive sign of strength. When you do relate to an issue, consider it an area in which you will need to find inner resources. Make use of this important guideline: *Every time you gain strength in your personal life you will be laying a solid foundation for mastering panic.*

Karen L. is a thirty-four-year-old mother of two who began experiencing anxiety at age seven. She can remember at that age running home from friends' houses because of overwhelming feelings of fear. Once back in her own room she felt momentary relief from those strange tensions but would cry alone on her bed. After several years of psychological treatment, she became free of these problems. Then, during her senior year in high school, her father died. For the next twelve months she withdrew into depression and rarely ventured outside her bedroom. The following year her family moved to another city. Within a few months, Karen began to have panic attacks, first in restaurants, then at movies and on trips.

Now, thirteen years later, Karen continues to experience panic, especially when traveling anywhere alone. Her physical discomfort includes rapid heartbeat, blurred vision, clenched jaws, weakness, numbness, shooting headache pains, chest pain, and physical imbalance. Although she can comfortably travel with a companion, she rarely makes commitments for activities with others for fear that she will have to cancel plans.

Undoubtedly there were many experiences in Karen's childhood that contributed to her susceptibility to panic. But more relevant to this chapter is how Karen's problems are supported by her current self-image. In the following pages you will hear how she feels inferior to her peers, how she constantly criticizes her own actions, how she seeks approval from others yet refuses to accept their compliments. She believes that she is socially inept, that she is not capable of carrying on a normal conversation with her women friends. And she is so afraid of her husband's anger that she placates him through concession after concession.

When we place Karen's trouble within the context of her current life we can see how it reflects a basic self-distrust. She doesn't believe she has what it takes to handle the adult world. Therefore, whenever life places a challenge in front of her, she naturally becomes afraid. Although quite uncomfortable and distressing, her panic attacks are only one part of her fear of being forced into adult responsibility.

As she recovers from agoraphobia, Karen will learn to face traveling alone. But she will also learn that she is a unique and important member of our world, deserving of respect from others and deserving of her own self-respect. She will find that if her marriage is a good one, her husband won't leave her just because she sticks up for her needs. And she will learn that she can survive losses, she can tolerate mistakes, and she doesn't need the approval of all others to feel OK about herself.

Sheryll W. is a forty-five-year-old housewife who has experienced agoraphobia for twenty-two years. Her greatest difficulties come when she begins to plan for some event, large or small. As she contemplates going shopping, entering a crowded place, or driving to the beach she begins to feel smothered, as if she can't breathe. She feels dizzy and nauseated, her heart rate increases, and her legs become weak. At the same time, her mind races through a series of fearful thoughts about the activity. If she decides to venture out, all she can think about is getting back home. After several hours of this anxious anticipation, Sheryll becomes physically and emotionally depleted and withdraws into her house for several days.

Sheryll became pregnant on her honeymoon, and the panic attacks started when her child was born. After the birth, Sheryll's husband worked seven days and nights a week while she remained home. Thus, her life was dramatically altered: from enjoying a carefree, single life, she became isolated at home alone every night. Then, three months later, the family was evicted when their rental house was sold. She thought this was more than she could handle. Sheryll became depressed and anxious. One day, while trying to locate an apartment, she started having chest pains and thought she was dying of a heart attack. Her mother rushed her to the hospital, where the doctor diagnosed the problem as "anxiety" and prescribed tranquilizers. From that time on her problem became progressively worse. She began having difficulty attending church. Before long she became fearful at the supermarket. Within a year she was housebound, too afraid even to step outside her front door. During the past seventeen years she has gone through phases of improvement followed by dramatic setbacks. Like many with agoraphobia, Sheryll has been evaluated again and again by physicians. She spent several years in psychotherapy, tried a number of medications and was in and out of a psychiatric hospital for two years. In addition to her agoraphobia, she has suffered several bouts of severe depression.

But agoraphobia is more than being afraid of powerful physical discomfort. It is also the way people view themselves and their role in this world. Sheryll describes herself as the worrier in her family. She is always preparing for the worst, always on guard. Her biggest daily fear is that her husband will abandon her, even though she has no information that supports this dread. In general, her life revolves around anxiously bracing herself for some loss. Her fear of losing control in the grocery store is symbolic of a deeper belief about her life: If I let go and enjoy myself, something bad will happen.

Sheryll talks about her childhood, about how she lived in fear, confusion, and secret emotional pain, always worried that her alcoholic father would seriously injure her mother during his frequent Saturday night beatings. She talks about how her mother dominated her life, took away her independence as a teenager, made decisions for her, and attempted to control her thinking.

Such experiences leave a young woman unprepared for the responsibilities of adulthood. As she overcomes agoraphobia, Sheryll will master many new skills. In addition, she'll develop a special sense of independence. As a child she had little choice but to be afraid of her father's violence and to follow the overprotective directives of her mother. Today, however, she will learn a new self-trust that gives her a sense of freedom, choice, and independence.

Donna B. is a forty-seven-year-old married woman with three children. She has had agoraphobia for twenty-one years. For many of those years her anxiety was overshadowed by prolonged episodes of severe depression. Her first anxiety attack came three months after the birth of her oldest child. Over the past ten years she has become completely housebound for about two months each year. During her worst episodes she is unable even to leave her bedroom without panicking.

She has been hospitalized several times for treatment of her depression, including thoughts of suicide. Her treatment, however, never involved extended psychotherapy. Instead, it was limited to medications and electroconvulsive therapy (ECT), a neurological treatment for severe depression. When used with discretion, as it is today, ECT can produce spectacular changes in some severe depressions, sometimes within a handful of sessions. However, Donna was given more than one hundred ECT treatments over seven years. It's possible that this contributes to her long-term memory loss.

Donna is most susceptible to panic during the two-week period before and after her monthly menstruation. In her panic attacks she becomes dizzy and has blurred vision, poor concentration, weak leg muscles, clammy hands and cold feet, nausea, and tight jaw muscles. She also experiences depersonalization—the feeling that her mind and body are separated, as though she is in a dream. Her thoughts turn to the fear of losing control, and she wants to run. "If I stay here, I'll faint . . . I'll humiliate myself . . . I'll be overwhelmed by these feelings." Even more frightening is the question, "Am I about to become housebound again?"

Donna speaks of childhood experiences that are relevant to her struggle with agoraphobia. She was the youngest of five children; the next youngest sibling was eight years old when she was born. When she was seven her father died in a car accident. Her mother then became reclusive: she stopped socializing, never dated, and never remarried. Donna withdrew as well. For the next five years she went to school, came home, and helped prepare supper while her mother was at work, then spent the rest of the evening in her bedroom.

During her teenage years Donna allowed her mother to dominate her life. She "never argued, never said no." In her eyes her mother had made great sacrifices, so if Donna ever thought about opposing her, her sense of guilt would stop her assertive actions. Her most important task was to please her mother, and the easiest way to do that was to give up her own decision-making power. Donna explains how this relationship generalized to others later in her life, how she learned to hide her own needs while trying to do what others wanted.

There are several reasons Donna puts on this facade. One is her long-standing fear of abandonment. After her father died, Donna's only relationship for years was with her mother. Possibly her thinking was, "As long as I'm good, she won't leave me." And how does she think she can be "good"? By ignoring her own needs while focusing attention on what would make others happy. And that is what Donna does to this day.

The best way to ignore our needs is to ignore our feelings, for our emotions guide a great many of our decisions. As a young girl Donna paid a high price for her desire to keep her mother's love: she stopped paying attention to her own feelings. After years of practice, she is no longer able to distinguish her different feelings and manage them.

Donna's struggle with panic is closely related to her fear of abandonment, her depression, her need to please others, and her suppression of her own desires and feelings. She will not win over panic without also facing these lifelong issues. Over time she will learn that adults live interdependently. Each of us has the right, even the responsibility, to express our emotions directly and to strive for our personal goals in life without fearing the repercussions of isolation and abandonment. Close, caring friends and relatives want to know our feelings, even if different from their own. It is only through openly and honestly sharing our authentic feelings and needs that we establish ourselves as unique, special human beings. As Donna learns to trust this sharing process, she will not allow trapped emotions to express themselves through the vehicle of panic.

Ann C. is a thirty-nine-year-old married woman with one child. She began to experience panic attacks at twenty, just one month before her wedding day. After returning to work from her honeymoon, she remained highly anxious throughout her day, with headaches and episodes of panic. With the encouragement of her family she finally began treatment with a psychiatrist, who also placed her on a tranquilizer. After several months of weekly sessions without improvement, Ann stopped all treatment.

When her son was born four years later, Ann began self-treating her panic by avoiding more and more situations. This solution helped reduce her anxious episodes but at the same time greatly diminished her freedom of travel. Today, twelve years later, Ann never drives outside of her town. Whenever she drives within town, she must first devise an "escape route" back to some safe location, such as a friend's house. She is able to travel alone, but usually enlists the companionship of her son, her husband, or her mother. Her greatest difficulties are staying at home alone at night, grocery shopping, and standing in lines.

But what about the rest of Ann's life? Her rigid perfectionism keeps her from enjoying most achievements. She also has difficulty sorting out her emotions. She fears that if she lets herself feel angry, she will become explosive, so she avoids it at all costs. And she goes to great lengths to prevent anyone from becoming mad at her.

She speaks of her overdependence on her husband and her mother, how they fight her battles for her, how they "have always bailed me out whenever I've had to do something that makes me anxious." Within this protective system, she can always run away from conflict. But every time she runs away she reinforces her belief that she is incapable of handling life as an independent adult.

In addition to taking control of anxiety attacks, Ann will learn how to take charge of her self-esteem and pride. Her belief in her own self-worth will be based on something other than perfectionism or the opinions of others. She will find, through experience, that she can handle her own emotions and can manage her conflicts with others. Some of the changes will come easily, like learning to say thank-you when someone compliments her (instead of rejecting the compliment with some self-deprecating comment). Other changes will take more time, since they are part of her deeper fear of abandonment. As Ann recovers she will be less and less troubled by her profound sense that to think, feel, and act for herself will cause her to lose everyone and everything she values in this world.

Dorothy P. was seventy-two years old when we met. She has experienced agoraphobia for the past fifty years, but hasn't had an anxiety attack in over thirty years. Long ago she learned that if she avoided all uncomfortable situations she could avoid panic, and that is just what she has done. She never travels outside the city limits, never drives a car, never stays home alone, or goes out alone. She sits in the aisle seat at the movie theater, walks out into the lobby several times during the show, and always leaves before the end of the movie. If she goes to a restaurant she sits next to the door and keeps an eye on the exit throughout the meal, as though her escape might be blocked at any moment. In other words, she never challenges her fears; she stays away from all things that might produce a sense of being trapped.

A brief review of Dorothy's early life shows how one's past can have a direct bearing on one's current susceptibility to the fear of panic. Her father died during World War I, when she was a young child. A few years later her mother remarried. Dorothy explains how her mother rarely left the house—she probably also had agoraphobia—and her stepfather did all the shopping. Her stepfather continually ridiculed her and her sisters and controlled and physically abused their mother. Her loving, caring mother eventually broke under the abusive hands of her stepfather. Dorothy developed the traits of a perfectionist at an early age so as not to give her stepfather any justifiable reason to attack her verbally. When she was fourteen their family doctor placed her on tranquilizers because of her anxiety.

At seventeen she married to escape from her home life. Her new husband was as strong-willed as her stepfather. To Dorothy this was an important trait, because while growing up she never learned how to think independently about her own needs. It was important to marry someone who would also take care of her.

But soon this relationship turned on her as well. After the birth of their second child, her husband's alcoholism flared. As he drank he became violent. When their new daughter was only three months old, he came home one night in a drunken rage. Dorothy ended up in the hospital with a fractured jaw and a concussion. With the help of the courts she pressed charges, became legally separated, and then divorced her husband.

But her problems didn't end. Her ex-husband began to appear at her house randomly during the day or night, sometimes breaking down a door or window to demand "visitation rights." Dorothy lived in constant, anxious fear of a sudden violent attack.

It was during this traumatic period in her life that Dorothy's panic began to surface. Returning home on the train after a day at the beach with her two children, she suddenly became overwhelmed with fear and the need to escape. Within a matter of two weeks she restricted her travels to within her hometown.

Dorothy explains how she married the second time not for love, but for security; how she never wanted to "cause trouble" by making demands of her children or her second husband. She kept herself from expressing angry feelings by thinking, "They're going to lock me up." In her mind she believed she could never be in control of her anger, that she'd be angry every day if she allowed it. In Chapter 7 you'll hear Dorothy say that she never drives a car for fear of completely losing control. "If there was a detour or if traffic backed up, I'd have to either get out and run or jam on the brakes, knock everyone down, knock the policeman down, go through red lights. . . ."

Dorothy's recovery from agoraphobia will depend on her willingness to face fears she has avoided for almost fifty years. Her central fear is not a fear of driving a car or being alone at home; it is the fear of her own emotions. She has a number of legitimate emotions that she has held inside year after year. She keeps them in check by scaring herself with exaggerated images of losing control.

Dorothy will not resolve this problem by herself. She will do it with the help of new friends and a supportive professional who will help her express her authentic emotions a little at a time. As she does this she will learn how her emotions can express her personal values and her self-esteem. She will begin to reassess her priorities with regard to personal relationships. Being protected by a strong individual will be less and less important as she learns to manage her own life. And the desire to be close to loving, active friends will slowly increase in value. While these changes are taking place, she will begin to face panic by gradually expanding her restricted limits.

Her first task, however, will be to stop verbally degrading herself. Dorothy's stepfather was wrong; she is not stupid, incapable, or worthless. The sooner she changes these personal beliefs, the sooner she can start taking control of panic.

"I've Always Felt Inferior"

When a person with agoraphobia also has low self-esteem, she is usually self-critical and places others above her in life. She may not take on a new challenge because she doubts her ability or competence. When looking back over her past she sees only a series of failures.

What's more, a person with low self-esteem will tend to think that other people see her in a similar light. "Who could possibly like me?" is the question in the back of her mind. Since she doubts people could like her for just being who she is, she will try to make people like her through her generosity and self-sacrifice.

The major problem with this approach is that she attempts to get others to appreciate her before she learns to like herself. If it really were true that other people needed to be persuaded to like her, the problem would not be so difficult. But she is her own worst critic; when someone says, "Good job!" she says in her mind, "No, it wasn't."

This is quite a painful process. So much time and worry is spent seeking the approval of others that the woman is actually out of control. How *other people* act toward her determines how she feels about herself.

KAREN: We lose our self-confidence. That's what agora-phobia does to us. We just don't deserve it. We're not good enough. We overcompensate because we're just not worthy.

I probably spend all my waking hours looking for approval, recognition, and attention. I think I've always felt inferior, thinking that everyone else can do better than me. I need someone to build me up constantly, which is bad because no one's going to do that.

Acceptance. That's my biggest issue. I am so criti-cal of myself. I'm never content with my performance. Even when I am complimented on something, I think, "That's just not my best." It's strange, but I think deep inside I hate myself—I really do.

Here, Donna discusses her current relationship with her mother. As she speaks I notice her eyes beginning to water and her face flushing with color.

DR. W.: There's that sadness again.
DONNA: No, it's resentment. Resentment that I've let myself be pushed around all my life. I've allowed it to happen. I never said no to my mother. Never. If I thought about it, I felt guilty. And the guilt was diffi-cult to deal with. Even today, she will constantly try to lay guilt on me—that she's all alone, I should spend more time with her, that other mothers and daugh-ters are so close. Well, I can't tolerate much of her.
DR. W.: This inability to say no to your mother—does that generalize into other relationships?

DONNA: Yes. I have always been a people pleaser. If you
wanted to go to a restaurant, you'd decide the restaurant and I would say, "Fine." I could hate the place,
but I would say, "Wonderful."

Karen speaks of needing acceptance and approval. Although
this is a natural need for all of us, she allows her entire life to
revolve around her fear of disapproval. At the same time she
says, "I'm never content with my performance." Before she can
believe that other people accept her, she must learn to accept
herself.

She explains that she continues to give to others because she
wants to make up for being "not good enough." Where did that
standard come from? What are her criteria for "good enough"?
For some reason, Karen has set standards for herself that she can't
meet, and that means she's not "worthy." Belief in one's self-worth
is essential to conquering panic.

Donna presents another dimension of low self-esteem. She
doesn't deserve to say yes to herself. She will say yes to everyone
else in her life; she reserves saying no for her own needs.

Here are five components of one typical belief system of a
person who won't say no to others:

1. I am not worth much as a human being.
2. Therefore, I'm lucky this person has stayed with me
   for so long.
3. I don't deserve all that this person has generously
   given.
4. I owe him or her a great deal.
5. Therefore, I would feel guilty if I refused this request.

This faulty line of reasoning is often supported by a second
set of beliefs:

1. I must not forget that I am not worth much as a human being.
2. If this person left me because I didn't keep pleasing him or her, then most likely I would end up alone in the world.
3. Not only would I be isolated and lonely, but I would not be capable of managing my life.
4. Therefore, I must forget myself and think of others at all times.

"I Can't Stand Making a Mistake"

The strongly self-critical person often demands perfection, but only of herself.

DR. W.: Do you feel as if you have to be perfect at everything you do?

DONNA: Oh, yes. In the sense that either I do it up to my expectations or I don't do it at all. I have a real problem being a perfectionist. I don't demand perfection of other people, only of myself. I'll always say to someone else, "That's fine! You did the best you could do," but I can't seem to apply that to myself. And I can't stand making a mistake. Doing paperwork, even if nobody knows that I make the mistake, and even if I correct it on the next line. I get this really frustrated feeling—it's just unacceptable to me.

DR. W.: Is there any other time that it gets in your way?

DONNA: Yes, in my hesitation to try things. I don't venture to try certain things for fear of making a mistake or not being perfect. I'd rather not do them at all.

Notice the significance of Donna's last statements. She is not speaking of hesitating to go shopping or move in a crowd. She is speaking of not attempting *any* new, creative tasks that might be pleasurable or rewarding, such as painting a picture or writing a poem. Some with agoraphobia, if they take time to notice, can see that they don't just avoid phobic situations; they avoid any chance of making a mistake—because to make a mistake is one more way for them to feel out of control. If they can't guarantee that an undertaking will be done perfectly, they will not even begin the task.

> ANN: I can't say, "Well, that's good enough." It might be a question of one little detail that nobody will notice. But anything that I do that reflects me, that I'll get praise for, I have to do perfectly. Somebody might see it and say, "Oh, isn't that beautiful! Oh, you're so talented. Isn't that nice!" But while they're telling me that, I don't believe them. I just kind of laugh it off. I say, "Oh, it's silly, you can do it. Anybody can do it." I always put it down. Or if I make something and there's something about it bothers me, I'll always point it out. I'll say, "See, I didn't do so well right there."

Ann works compulsively at any task that might bring praise from others. After tremendous effort, she finally receives her deserved acknowledgment. Even at the exact moment the person is speaking, Ann is discounting the compliment in her own mind. And as if that weren't enough, she then explains to her friend that the praise was undeserved, since there was a flaw in the workmanship.

Can you imagine a carpenter spending all weekend remodeling his kitchen, then on Sunday night taking a sledgehammer to his handiwork? How about an account manager spending all day generating a report, then at five o'clock placing it in the shredder? Think of the carpenter or account manager repeating that same procedure every week, and now you are getting the picture of someone with agoraphobia. People like Donna and Ann make a career out of working toward self-worth, then never accepting it. It is an exhausting cycle.

Strong self-esteem is important as you begin to control panic. When you start to believe in your own worth, then you can start to believe that panic is standing in the way of an important person—you. You will feel more energy to push through setbacks and tough times. You will devote more attention to your own needs and less attention to having to please others.

Here are some questions to reflect on:

- Am I devastated by others' criticisms?
- Do I tend to point out all my mistakes to myself and others?
- Do I accept compliments? Do I really believe people when they speak well of me or my accomplishments?
- Do I need to do everything perfectly? Can I accept my mistakes?
- If I can't do something perfectly, do I avoid it?
- Do I have trouble setting limits on how much I give to others?
- Do I have trouble setting limits on any projects I undertake?
- Do I hesitate to try new tasks for fear I will fail?
- Do I consider mistakes to mean the same thing as failure?
- Am I constantly watching and monitoring myself? Do I evaluate my every move?
- Do I consider everything that I do to be of great significance? Or, do I use good judgment to determine the difference between small and large tasks, significant and insignificant projects?
- How many times have I said yes to myself this week? This year?

Your answers to these questions will indicate how much you withhold support from yourself and how hard you work at gaining the support of people around you.

If your self-esteem could use some strengthening, here are a few guidelines to help you on your way:

- Refrain from calling yourself names or putting yourself down for your mistakes. Life is hard enough. No one deserves to be humiliated, even silently by themselves.
- Never stop setting goals and standards for yourself, only bring them within reach. Success breeds success.
- Set a small enough goal, work to reach it, praise yourself for your effort, then set yourself a new reachable goal.
- When someone compliments you, be a sponge; absorb the compliment, believe it, feel it.
- When someone criticizes you, don't swallow it whole. Chew on it to see if you can learn anything for next time. Spit out any name-calling and hostility. Digest only what you believe is beneficial.
- Reevaluate your self-expectations. Make certain that they are based on your own belief system, what you think is good and right today. Do not allow beliefs taught years ago to rule your life without questioning them. Take control of your expectations and you will have control of your self-esteem.
- Find ways to say yes to yourself every day of your life. If you are unwilling to say yes to yourself, why should anyone else?

"But if I Didn't Have Him . . ."

Self-doubt can produce a multitude of questions in all parts of your life. At a party, for example: "Will I be able to stay the whole time? Will I embarrass myself? Will it get worse? Will anybody see me?" Those same types of doubting questions can be found elsewhere in an individual's life, and nowhere will self-doubt have a more dramatic effect than in the realm of personal relationships.

Consider, for example, a woman who has an underlying belief that she is inherently a weak person. "If I honestly believe that I am incapable of caring for myself, then I have to find someone in my life who will protect me. I might hate being dependent, I might detest my subservience to another human being, but those feelings will never be stronger than my fear of going it alone. If I believe I will be helpless if left alone, my basic survival is at stake. All other considerations take on lesser importance; I must survive. Therefore I must keep people around me, at whatever cost."

This is a crucial issue in the understanding of panic. Our belief systems will always overpower any other thoughts or emotions. Many of these beliefs were adopted years ago and are outside our conscious awareness. This is what is so confusing for those with agoraphobia. They really would love not to have to depend on others; they want independence more than almost anything else in the world. But their belief systems tell them that they won't survive without a strong person next to them. Keeping this significant conflict in mind, see how it has caused so much pain in these women's lives.

DOROTHY: When I met my second husband, something should have gone off in my head, I should have known that he was not going to be a friend. We had no common interests, we had nothing to talk about. Something told me—I don't know what it was—that I was going to be sick and unable to work; I was going to need a roof over my head. I had had it up to here trying to make ends meet. I was really wanting security. I didn't love him, not at all.

Dorothy made a major life decision based on fear. In order to gain security, she surrendered love, happiness, and companionship.

KAREN: I think I don't want to grow up—that's what I really feel. I just don't want to admit it. I don't want to be thirty-four, with two children; I don't want my responsibilities. I know that I can get rid of agoraphobia tomorrow, but then where do I go? I'm not ready for the adult world. I don't know how to act. I mean, I don't know how to pull up in people's driveways and talk to them.

ELIZABETH (to Karen, in a group therapy session): One night when we came out of here, you were rushing to go to your husband, and I wanted to talk to you for a minute. Your husband was outside and you said, "If I keep him waiting for too long, he'll get mad. If he sees me crying, he'll get mad and say, 'You can't come here anymore.'" And I say, "The hell with him, the hell with him!" You can use us, the hell with him. Lean on us, that's what a support group is for.

KAREN: You're right, you're right. I know that. It's a nightmare the way it is now. But I don't know how much of a nightmare it would be if I didn't have him.

ELIZABETH (still angry): So therefore you would rather do everything his way?

KAREN: I get up in the morning and I say, "How low do you have to lie? I mean, how low does someone like me have to go? How long will I let him treat me this way?" But to turn around and say, "Knock it off, I want to be my own person"—I can't say that to my husband. I need him too badly.

Karen says that she doesn't want to grow up. That is probably based on her belief that she is not capable of handling her responsibilities. She worried so much about failing as a mother that she gave her entire attention to her children. She monitored her every move and left no time for her own pleasures. She now believes that the world has passed her by, that she no longer knows how to communicate with her peers.

Her belief that she is incapable is so strong that she allows herself to be dominated by her husband. She hates what she is doing to herself. And I am sure some of her friends have said, "If you hate it so much, why don't you change it?" But, as Karen says, she believes she can't, that she is not capable of independence. Therefore, her actions continue to lower her self-esteem. She fears the loss of her husband's support because she believes she cannot survive without him.

KAREN: When I need to get my daughter to the doctor for a checkup or I need to shop for new clothes, I have to say to my husband, "Three weeks from Saturday, would you take me to the mall?" And I have to build him up. I think, "No, I'd better not antagonize him because he'll say, 'OK, we're not going.'" What a way to live! I have no control over my own life.

ANN: My mother will still do my fighting for me, and I'm thirty-nine years old. My husband does a lot for me, too. He's the "take charge" kind of person. So I have these two people that have always bailed me out when I've had to do something that makes me anxious. Even now, if I go to a group meeting my husband will say, "What time are you going to be home?" And if I'm a little bit late, he gets upset. I always say I'm his oldest child, because he treats me like a child in a lot of ways. But I let him treat me like a child; I don't assert myself with him. It doesn't seem worth it. I'm just happy to go along like this. My husband and my mother are always around to help me with this, to help me with that. I don't want to lose them but, deep down inside, I know that it's wrong. Still, I fear what will happen if I start to get really independent.

As you may be starting to sense, if a person feels as though she is incapable of managing the demands of the world, she will search out someone who can manage them for her. Perhaps she is skilled at giving to others, being kind and sensitive, but feels unable to stand up for herself when necessary. Within the logic of that belief system, she believes that she would be smart to marry a man who is powerful, dominant, and controlling. Together they make a whole person, one who can be kind, compassionate, and giving, and also strong and forceful if need be.

Unfortunately, they are *two* people, not one. This has caused many a painful marriage. They may stay together because they satisfy certain basic needs (simply put, he remains dominant and receives nurturing while she feels protected). But other needs go unmet or get stifled, because each person behaves completely differently. He controls and dominates, she surrenders and submits. They don't have a common, shared relationship between two equals. It is very difficult for them to have fun together, to solve problems together, to plan the future together.

"If I Stop Worrying, Something Bad Will Happen"

Over time, our roles and self-perceptions begin to solidify within our relationships. In the above example, Ann sees herself as always the child, both with her mother and with her husband. Sheryll sees herself as the worrier.

SHERYLL: Nothing ever bothers my husband. And my kids take after him. Nothing ever gets on his nerves. Everything's very easy for them.

DR. W: So what role does that leave you?

SHERYLL: I do all the worrying. Somebody's got to worry in my family! [Laughs.]

DR. W: Or what would happen?

SHERYLL: I've never thought of the consequences. Nothing would get done. All my husband cares about is his tennis.

DR. W.: "I have to keep worrying about the kids, because if I don't . . ."? Fill in the blank, Sheryll.

SHERYLL: Well, I'm afraid something will happen if I stop worrying about this, that, and the other thing. If I relax and take it easy, if I stop worrying, something bad will happen. Does that make sense? I'm always prepared. I've been married twenty-three years. And still, every night when my husband walks through the door, I wait for him to say, "Sheryll, I've found somebody else." This is how I live.

DR. W.: "I'm always on guard . . ."

SHERYLL: I'm always on guard, you'd better believe it.

Sheryll first states that she must worry or nothing would get done in her home. But with just a little prodding, she reveals a deeper, more significant concern. She expresses a basic fear of something bad happening to her, especially the fear of being abandoned. It is not a minor fear; Sheryll thinks about it every day. But it is an irrational fear, one based on an internal belief system rather than any real evidence. She tells me that her husband has given her no reason to doubt his commitment to the marriage.

But she does give us an important piece of information, something that I doubt she understood at the time she said it. It is as though she has a magical strategy to prevent anything bad from happening. Her belief is, "As long as I keep worrying, as long as I remain tense and on guard, nothing bad will happen. If I relax and take it easy, if I stop worrying . . ." This is exactly the same feeling that a person has about panic attacks. She remains tense in anticipation of a negative experience (at a store, in a car, or in a crowd). She remains on guard, expecting the worst. For Sheryll and other panic-prone people, that fear epitomizes the way they think about their life in general.

Looking back over Sheryll's therapy we were able to see this thought pattern more clearly. The interview you just read took place during our tenth session. Prior to that I had taught Sheryll a relaxation process (which you will find in Chapter 16). She was petrified at the thought of listening to the exercise on an audio-tape. "I *can't* relax," she said. I instructed her to do some household chore, like her ironing, while playing the tape on low volume in the background, just as a way to get used to the sound. She was so afraid of the concept of relaxation that she would not take the risk. At that point, relaxation meant loss of control.

After this tenth session, I learned that her unconscious fear was long-standing and of a much stronger nature. She feared great harm or loss if she let go of her tension and worry. Her tension was her protection. Unfortunately, this belief was causing her great discomfort in her current life. But in her mind, her worry and tension seemed to be working, because she had averted any trouble. Since she always remained tense, she assumed her method of self-protection was successful. You may remember the old joke of the man who constantly paces around the outside of his house to keep away the tigers. "There aren't any tigers loose around here," exclaims his neighbor. "See how well it works," responds the man. The use of physical as well as psychological tension to guard against mistakes or harm takes this same strategy. Even to experiment with relaxing holds too many risks.

"I Am Deathly Afraid of That Anger"

There are few people who could say that they enjoy conflicts. Most people feel somewhat uncomfortable before, during, or after an argument. But for many with agoraphobia, conflicts are to be avoided like the plague.

> ANN: Last winter I was hemmed in in a parking space downtown. Someone parked illegally behind me, and I became livid. It was very cold and I had one child with me. Just driving into town with my children was a big step, because I was really feeling housebound at the time. Well, I came out and said, "How am I going to get out of this space? Look at that jerk parked there."
>
> It started welling up in me—the anger. I thought that I should stay and give him a piece of my mind, that I should call the cops because he'd parked illegally. Then all I could think about was getting out of there, getting the heck out of there and getting home. I didn't want to confront this. I didn't want this person to come out because I would have had to get mad and I wasn't sure what that would do to me.
>
> DR. W.: So you'd start to have those feelings about getting mad, and you even had the image of getting angry at the person. At the same time you'd be thinking, "Let me get away from it."
>
> ANN: Yes, but not all the time, because I can get mad, too. But that happened to be a particularly sensitive week, when I was feeling a lot of panic. I was highly sensitized.

Women such as Ann will expend much energy to avoid a confrontation because it might lead to a separation or loss of relationship. They can also fear their own intense emotions, such as anger. Ann did not want to confront the driver of that car, "because I would have had to get mad and I wasn't sure what that would do to me." What did she fear? That she would lose control of her feelings in a dangerous way. Listen to how Donna reflects that same fear.

DONNA: I've had an awfully hard time with anger. I have trouble sorting out my emotions. Sometimes I think my feelings get tangled into a big ball. I don't know if I'm mad, or what.

I really don't get mad at all. And if I do, I keep it all in. I mean, I don't direct it at anything. I suppose I'm directing it at myself and just running away from it.

My husband never knows what I'm feeling. I never share negative feelings. I'm one of those people who talks positively and feels negatively. And I always play that game. I tell people what I judge they want to hear. If I feel angry, they never hear about it—I never show it. I don't even think I give nonverbal cues for anger. A person would have to be very in tune to me to see a nonverbal. I just suppress a lot of stuff. And I think the reason isn't so much that I don't want to show I am angry as that I never really feel just anger, I feel rage. And I am deathly afraid of losing control of that anger, of hurting somebody. Consequently, it is unusual for me to even raise my voice in the house. When I yell at the kids, they move, because I so seldom do it.

DR. W.: So your anger has to evolve to a bigger level before you even begin to notice it yourself.

DONNA: Yes, I have to feel it to an extreme. And then I sometimes don't know exactly what I'm feeling. When I feel anger and rage it's usually mixed with self-pity. When I feel fear, it's more terror than fear.

DOROTHY: I was too lenient with the kids, and I'm still too lenient with my husband. If he says something, I think to myself, "Why cause trouble? Why have an argument? I'll just let it go." But once in a blue moon, I hit the roof.

DR. W.: And what would happen if you did that more often?

DOROTHY: Well, I'd be doing it every day of the week. Why bother getting upset over something that's not going to change? My fear is that they're going to lock me up.

Donna and Dorothy speak of holding in their emotions. Whenever we hold on to something tightly, we feel tension. Try physically holding your fist in a tight squeeze for one minute, and you'll experience the amount of psychic energy we must use to hold in our secret emotions. It is exhausting physically and emotionally.

To incorporate our emotions into our lives in a beneficial way, it is important to do three things:

1. Notice what emotion you are feeling.
2. Respect that emotion as a legitimate expression of who you are and what you value as a human being.
3. Take care of that emotion in some manner. Simply acknowledging the presence of a feeling inside you and permitting it to exist can sometimes be enough. If the emotion is in response to another person, you may need to express it directly to the person who stimulated your reaction. In still other situations it may be more beneficial for you to express your emotion to a more objective and supportive listener instead of the person to whom you are reacting.

Your values and your emotions are the two essential ingredients that distinguish you as a unique individual. When you cut other people off from knowing your values and emotions or if you only present the values and emotions you think they want to see, then you do yourself and them a disservice. You don't give people a chance to treat your true self with respect. You do the same thing when you cut yourself off from knowing your feelings. You don't respect your rights and your values as a human being.

In addition, when you refuse to pay attention to your milder emotions, they tend to grow stronger to be heard. Everyone knows what it's like to be in a noisy environment calling out someone's name. "John?" (in a normal tone). No answer. "John?" (a little louder). Not even a turn of the head. "JOHN?!" you yell with force, finally grabbing his attention. John will probably jump, startled.

Your emotions work the same way. As you ignore them, they grow and grow. Once they are so big that you can't ignore them, they scare you instead. That's what Donna's just told us—her fear turns into "terror."

"And He Never Came Back"

You've been reading about several traits that are sometimes present in the panic-prone personality: low self-esteem, self-criticism and self-doubt, worrying, the need to do every task perfectly, the need to please others, and the fear of anger or conflicts. These characteristics do not develop after panic begins; typically they begin long before. The primary decisions we make about our future, most of the beliefs we hold, and the ways we view ourselves and our world—all these seem to be shaped between birth and our teenage years, so our personal histories can tell us a great deal about our current lives.

When we are born into this world, we are completely helpless and vulnerable. We are dependent on our parents for our every need, our very survival. The process of development from birth to late adolescence is a progressive maturing—physically, emotionally, intellectually, and socially. Critical to that maturing is learning independence—thinking for ourselves, trusting our instincts, setting personal goals, having confidence in our own abilities, and being capable of independent living.

In normal development, by the time a child is two years old she has begun to strike out on her own by opposing her parents through a broad range of "terrible twos" maneuvers and by learning to feed herself. By age six, she has learned that it is OK to disagree, to speak up and to ask questions. By the time the normally developed child is eleven years old, her interactions with her peer group have evolved to a sophisticated level. She is skilled at arguing, competing, achieving, and negotiating. By sixteen, the teenager is in the process of adopting a comfortable sexual identity and self-image. She has learned to be assertive and to initiate activities while taking adult responsibility for many of her actions. By young adulthood, the woman has acquired a sense of self-worth. She can take risks and take time for her own activities, even if they conflict with the activities of others.

As you can see, achieving a sense of independence is a gradual, step-by-step developmental process, equal in intensity and importance to our physical growth during those same eighteen years. None of us had perfect parents, nor can any of us *be* perfect as parents. It is not beneficial to blame anyone for what happened in the past. Every parent does the best that he or she can. Very few parents purposely hurt their children. Nonetheless, if we fail to achieve certain developmental tasks when we are young, our ability to experience independence as adults will be restricted.

All of us have the ability to overcome any developmental limitations. We have the power now, as adults, to identify the strengths we are missing and to train ourselves in independent thinking, feeling, and living. Childhood experiences are not excuses for our adult difficulties.

I look to the past with my clients for one primary reason: to identify what new learning is needed. This looking back helps my clients understand certain current beliefs in light of past experiences. However, studying the past does not in itself change anything. Only positive action today changes how we think, feel, or act.

Some of my clients had quite traumatic experiences in their childhood. I share their stories with you because they can best illustrate how some unconscious learning takes place. I do not intend to imply that all those with agoraphobia have had unhappy childhoods, because I don't believe this to be true. I do want to suggest that some beliefs may be irrational, acquired unconsciously. Many lessons we receive during our lifetimes are quite subtle. But nonetheless they shape our belief systems, and what we believe strongly determines how we act.

DONNA: My father died when I was seven. And I don't really remember the next five years of my life. I spent a lot of time in my bedroom during those five years. I would go to school, come home, help out around the house, and then I would go upstairs and listen to the radio.

I was one of five kids, but when I was born, my brothers and sisters were much older than me. They were already in junior high school. So it was really just my mother and I. She never socialized or dated any other men and never remarried. She worked very hard, was very loving and giving.

DOROTHY: My father joined the service during the war. And he never came back—he was killed. I can remember the day we heard of his death. I think maybe that's when it started. From that point on my mother gave up her life for us.

Both of these women experienced a significant loss during childhood. Both Donna and Dorothy have a traumatic scene etched in their minds: one in which their fathers disappeared and never returned. At seven years old, Donna was given no explanation of death or of how to manage her feelings in response to death. She became depressed and remained that way for many years, withdrawing from the world and feeling a void.

She now has no memories of those years, but we can presume that she had great difficulty understanding or expressing her emotions, in part because of this early childhood experience.

While we are children, our parents serve as our models of how to act in life. Dorothy's mother withdrew from the world after Dorothy's father died. She watched her mother become isolated, stop taking care of herself, and rarely leave the home. Donna's mother made the same decision. Both girls watched their mothers surrender their personal lives while continuing to give to their children.

Four issues are significant to our understanding of childhood learnings:

1. Experiencing the loss of a significant person is highly traumatic to a child, who can also become confused as to why the person left. Death, separation, and divorce can lead a child to wonder, "Did I cause that?" The child may become fearful of her actions, not being sure which behaviors were "wrong." According to a child's logic, if you can be abandoned once, you can be abandoned again. That is a terribly frightening thought. A child might make a variety of decisions to avoid another loss or separation. One is to resolve not to get close to anyone else, to prevent further hurt. Another is to be very good, not to make waves, because if you are bad, people might leave you. These are examples of unconscious decisions that can remain in place into adulthood. But this store of beliefs influences many decisions in adulthood. It can lead the person to resolve, "I'd better keep pleasing the people around me, or I'll be left alone."

2. When one parent leaves or dies, the child can develop a strong attachment to the remaining parent. That attachment can become a powerful unconscious force which plays havoc with the person's future life. As adults we have responsibilities that require us to think, feel, and act independently. With unresolved attachments, we can suffer great internal conflict.

Many of my clients speak of their resentment of parents who are too close to them emotionally or who attempt to run their lives, or a spouse who tries to dominate them. At the same time, they feel incapable of setting limits on the relationship and are unable to bring about a separation as adults. They make statements such as "I'm angry about how my mother treats me, and yet she is my closest friend. I don't know what I would do without her."

3. Experiencing a loss produces a great many emotions. For a child, it can be the first time she has felt so many feelings so intensely: sadness, fear, surprise, shock, even anger. She will probably feel confused and overwhelmed by these new sensations. Unless special care is taken, it is possible she will never sort out those feelings. Donna, for example, remained swallowed up by that confusion as she began treatment some thirty years later.

4. When we are young, our parents or guardians constitute our entire world. This is the concept of "modeling." They probably model 90 percent of all our learned behaviors. We learn, by observing their actions, how to share our feelings of love and affection, how to solve problems, how to communicate with others, how to respect ourselves, how to face the world. Both Donna and Dorothy watched their mothers become socially isolated and withdrawn. What they did not see was a woman who had self-pride and self-esteem, who looked on life as a challenge. At the same time, though, both received a great deal of love and affection from their mothers. This, I am sure, was a positive, nourishing experience, which they remember and appreciate to this day. No one's childhood is all bad or all good.

DONNA: My mother went out to work after my father died, though she had never worked before in her life. I felt I was a burden, so I never made waves. I never gave her any aggravation. I always did what I could do around the house to help out. I was very grateful that we were able to keep the house that I grew up in, that we didn't have to move, change our environment.

DR. W.: What makes you think she thought you were a burden?

DONNA: The fact that she had to go out to work in order to maintain that house, that she had never worked and so forth.

DR. W.: So this was something that you decided on your own, as opposed to any cues that she was giving you?

DONNA: I think so. I don't really remember any particular cues.

Here Donna describes her belief (that she was a burden) and her decision (not to make waves) based on that belief. Notice that her belief was not based on anything that her mother did or said. She also felt grateful that nothing else was taken from her after her father died. She was careful to be good, so that her mother wouldn't leave her also. As an adult, Donna has incorporated these early childhood decisions into all of her relationships. She hides her needs if they might conflict with the needs of others and works hard to please those around her. Even with her closest friends, she smiles on the outside when she is actually feeling sad or hurt. It is as though the same childhood fears continue to plague her: "If I express my needs, I'll be too much of a burden and others will abandon me."

"I Lived in Fear That Something Would Happen"

DR. W.: Tell me more about what it was like in your home.

SHERYLL: Oh, Saturday nights I'd wake up and my father would be beating my mother up and . . . oh, I don't know . . . [Voice trails off. She looks down at the floor.]

DR. W.: You don't want to talk about it.

SHERYLL: It was tension. What else can I tell you? It just stunk. I used to be mad because other families seemed so intact, and I had to put up with this. There was always this fear. I guess I lived in fear that my father would do something to my mother. Don't get me wrong, it was weekends that he was really frightening. Other than that, he'd put up with a lot of garbage from her. She was an aggressive woman in her own way.

I didn't feel secure in the house. I always felt that something bad would happen, that one Saturday night, something was going to happen. The situation was at its worst during my teens. Maybe going to school and being a cheerleader and being in clubs was my way of blocking all this out. I don't know.

Long before Sheryll developed agoraphobia, she lived in fear. She had no control over her environment. She had reason to be afraid that "something bad was going to happen," since her father physically abused her mother. But it was not something that she could prevent as a young girl. Her only option was to avoid the situation, to be outside of the home as much as possible.

Notice how this is similar to the response someone with panic has toward fearful situations: to worry about something bad happening over which one has no control and to avoid the situation as much as possible. This early life experience provided Sheryll's first lesson in such behavior.

SHERYLL: I was very confused as a child. Sometimes I wished that my father would leave or my mother would pull herself together. It was very difficult. But on the outside, I always acted as if everything was fine. People on the outside would never know there was anything going on in the house.

Sheryll made a generous, unselfish decision to protect her family's secret. She hid her feelings from all her friends so they wouldn't discover the problems within her household. But she did this to her own personal detriment. She pretended to be a happy-go-lucky, active child on the outside, while on the inside she was sad, confused, tense, and scared. Since no one knew of her emotional pain, no one could respond to it in a caring manner. Sheryll decided at a young age to withhold her emotions. This decision and all its repercussions served as the foundation of many personal difficulties later in life.

KAREN: I have suffered from anxiety since the age of eight. I can remember actually having to run home because of overwhelming feelings that I had, but couldn't logically understand at the age and mentality of five. And from that point on, I was labeled an emotionally disturbed child. I was also asthmatic. I coped with it as best I could. I just accepted it, and if I didn't feel well while over at a friend's house (this is at the age of eight), I'd just go home. I always knew what I had to do. And then when I got home I'd feel relief. But I'd go in my room and cry; I'd have deep depression.

In grammar school and in junior high school, I always had a lot going for me. Then, when I was a teenager, I went to an analyst at some type of clinic because my mother thought I was depressed.

DR. W.: Why?

KAREN: As I look back on it I can remember that I spent a lot of time in my room—one whole year, in fact. And I had no goals, no achievements, no ambition.

DR. W.: When was that?

KAREN: Right at the time that my father died. I was a senior in high school. During that year after my father died I'd shut myself in my room. I just wanted time out, wanted my own time. And I caused my own depression, I'm sure. In fact, when I was depressed, I had no anxiety, I just secluded myself from everybody.

I remember that my first anxiety attack came when we were moving. I left the place where I had grown up. My mother had remarried, and we were moving to another state. And I had to leave my boyfriend. All this was happening at once. Important things—my house, my security. . .

DR. W.: How old were you then?

KAREN: Eighteen. And shortly after that I started having my spells. In restaurants, movies, theaters, on ski trips.

In this brief exchange, Karen describes three patterns that are common in some with agoraphobia.

1. She had a long-standing tendency toward anxiety.
2. She also suffered bouts of depression. In fact, her year of being housebound was more likely a depressive reaction to her father's death than it was a sign of agoraphobia.
3. Her panic attacks began during the time when her mother remarried and she had to move away from many important people and things in her life. This fits the pattern we have seen so far: Agoraphobia tends to manifest itself during a stressful period in the person's life.

Karen, Donna, and Dorothy reflect the histories of many women who suffer from agoraphobia. They have difficulty coping with separation, not just in childhood but throughout their lives. As adults, developing an independence from their parents or choosing to separate from an unhealthy marriage can produce feelings of overwhelming anxiety. Even though they may intellectually believe that a change is needed in the relationship, psychologically the task feels untenable. Karen's extreme reactions to her father's death and to the family's cross-country move are examples. This single issue can place a powerful roadblock in the way of recovery.

"So I Allowed Her to Dominate Me"

DONNA: When I got married, I had absolutely nothing to do with the wedding. I didn't pick out the gown, I didn't pick out my maid of honor. My mother wanted a particular girl and that was it. I was always trying to please her, because I felt that she had sacrificed for me. And so I allowed her to dominate.

SHERYLL: My mother has always been a very domineering woman. She wants to control the world. She's got to be in control at all times. When I was a teenager I was never allowed to do anything; she used to do everything for me. I never had any independence. She tells me that this is because she was the youngest of nine and had to do everything in her family. Well, she shouldn't take it out on me!

From those brief excerpts we observe that neither Donna nor Sheryll developed independent thinking and behavior during their teens. Regardless of the reason, they left their developmental years lacking an essential skill. Both of them has suffered greatly from that deficit.

To conquer panic, both of them must learn now what they should have learned then. If they fail to develop independence of thought, feeling, and action, they will remain trapped by their fear, hesitation to act, and self-doubt.

DOROTHY: My stepfather, no matter what we did, always bossed us. We never could do anything on our own. If we did one thing we were "stupid," if we did another we were "wrong." My mother was phobic, I guess, because he took charge of everything. He did the food shopping, my mother stayed home. He bossed my mother, he bossed me. He meant well, I'm sure he did, because we had a very good life, materially. But as I got older, I used to hear her crying a lot in bed.

My stepfather had to be right. She did try to fight him; as a child I remember them arguing about different things. But if they didn't go his way, he'd hit her. My mother was once lovely and strong. She ended up having a nervous breakdown. She's a nothing now, she just takes pills.

My mother would allow him to boss us. She'd say, "Just do it. Make him happy." In other words, we never had our own minds. We couldn't say, "I'm doing this because I want to do it." After a while, I think it was ingrained in me. I was a perfectionist even as a child. I wanted everything just so. And I worried about everything. They called me "anxious." I was more of an emotional type. At fourteen the doctor put me on a tranquilizer. I married my husband at seventeen to get away from the place. He was as strong as my stepfather, he also had control. So it's as if I never got the chance to find my own way.

These passages from Dorothy's session contain a wealth of information about her limitations today. First, Dorothy learned from her mother's modeling. It appears that her mother, too, was trapped by agoraphobia. Her world was no larger than the walls of her house. Simply *observing* the significant people and events around us in childhood provides us with a great many of our beliefs. Dorothy also watched her mother attempt to stand up to her stepfather—and fail. Standing up for what she thought was right produced not only physical pain but humiliation as well. Independent thinking or acting became associated with discomfort, over and over again. In that setting it was natural, even smart, for Dorothy to become passive and dependent.

She made two other decisions in attempting to cope at home. She became a perfectionist, and she worried about everything. Could her belief have been, "Maybe if I do things perfectly, he'll stop criticizing me?" Did she become anxious because she never knew what bad thing would happen next? "How will he react if I do this?" No matter what she did, her stepfather would never let her have control. In that setting, attempting to avoid his criticism may have been her best move.

The problem is that Dorothy's coping strategies as a child—to be passive, dependent, worried, and perfectionistic—became unconscious patterns that she continues to use today, even though the situation that made these strategies necessary is no longer present. In order to change, she will have to experience a new trust in the benefits of activity, independence, and an acceptance of mistakes.

The lessons we learn don't necessarily come from major, traumatic experiences; they can come from subtle influences, as illustrated by these comments from Helen, another client with agoraphobia: "I was an only child, and I always wanted to please my father, I think. If I was doing anything wrong, he never hit or scolded me or yelled. But he'd give me a look—that was all it took. My mother was a very passive person. She'd hold the peace at all costs, and I think I always wanted that, too—peace at all costs." Regardless of what actually took place in the home, it is the child's belief about the events that determines her current behavior. We are not run by our past, we are run by our learned beliefs. Helen watched her mother "hold the peace at all costs" by being a quiet, undemanding wife who would never argue. She also experienced a loving family and observed a happy marriage between her father and mother. One belief Helen adopted was that "keeping the peace" would produce a happy marriage, and she decided to follow that rule in her adult life.

Coping in the Present

The experience of panic in someone with agoraphobia is the physical manifestation of a complex constellation within the personality. Certainly a great many people in the world suffer through traumatic events, including the death of a parent or physical brutality. Even more people have experienced stressful periods during their lives that have produced brief episodes of anxiety and panic. All of us go through times of self-doubt and self-criticism, of wanting to please others, and of avoiding conflicts.

So what causes agoraphobia? Just as with most other psychological problems, we are not certain and probably never will be. The understanding of personality cannot be an absolute science. However, the patterns illustrated in this chapter reflect some of the common experiences of the present and the past that shape and support the panic-prone personality of someone with agoraphobia.

There is no going back to fix the past. There is no way to get today the things you failed to receive when you were younger. What is done is done. But, fortunately, knowing the causes of agoraphobia is a different issue than knowing how to cure it. Panic is maintained by our current beliefs and attitudes, our current emotions, and our current behaviors. These three parts of us *are* changeable, regardless of our past.

The self-help section of this book—Chapters 10 through 18— takes into account the many issues facing people with agoraphobia. Most important, they reflect my firm conviction that by attending to current beliefs, emotions, and actions one can overcome any obstacles in one's way.

However, one difference between people with agoraphobia and other panic-prone persons is that those with agoraphobia tend to feel stuck and have a sense that, "I'll never change." So many variables come into play during the treatment of this disorder; it's almost as though the moment of panic is like the tip of an iceberg.

If you have agoraphobia and you struggle to apply the skills within this book, you'll be wise to turn to a mental health professional to help guide you along the way. If you need my help in finding one, write me at rrw@med.unc.edu.

CHAPTER 5

Four Complicating Problems

There are four specific problems that can complicate the diagnosis and treatment of panic. The symptoms of panic closely resemble those of premenstrual syndrome and hypoglycemia. This can cause some difficulties in diagnosis. An incorrect diagnosis can delay appropriate treatment for some sufferers. Depression and alcoholism greatly disrupt the treatment process by lowering motivation and by contributing additional serious problems to an already complex picture.

Premenstrual Syndrome

Premenstrual syndrome (PMS), and its more severe form of premenstrual dysphoric disorder (PMDD), is the occurrence of a wide variety of physical and psychological symptoms in women during the days prior to menstruation. Studies have found that 30 to 95 percent of all healthy females may experience a premenstrual increase in depression, irritability, and anxiety in addition to physical discomfort, even though they don't reach the level of symptoms for a diagnosis of PMS or PMDD.

A woman suffering from PMS experiences moderate to severe emotional and/or physical symptoms, which may begin up to fourteen days before menstruation, but usually start five to seven days prior. The discomfort comes in almost every monthly cycle and only during the premenstrual phase. The symptoms disappear during the week after menstruation begins.

The menstrual cycle is one of the most complex functions of the body. Despite fifty years of research, we do not fully understand its process. There is no known cause of PMS that has been substantiated by large-scale research findings. No one treatment has achieved solid support, either. We can now say, however, that it is a physical, not psychological, disorder.

Since the possible kinds of symptoms are so numerous and can vary dramatically among women, I will present here only the psychological and behavioral symptoms that frequently occur during the premenstrual phase. Discuss with your physician if your symptoms are so severe that they seriously disrupt your life and if you have four or more of these sets of symptoms:

- Irritability, hostility, anger, "short fuse"
- Tenseness, restlessness, jitters, upset, nervousness, inability to relax
- Decreased efficiency, fatigue
- Depression, crying, spontaneous mood swings
- Poor coordination, clumsiness, proneness to accidents
- Distractibility, confusion, forgetfulness, difficulty with concentration
- Change in eating habits, usually cravings and overeating
- Increase or decrease in sexual desire

Although most women with PMS suffer both physical and psychological symptoms, the psychological symptoms can be the more devastating. PMS is one of several problems described in this book that often goes undiagnosed; since so many of its symptoms are psychological, the women, their families, and health professionals can dismiss it as "all in the head." Failure to receive a proper and early diagnosis can greatly complicate the problem.

We know that stress has a direct effect on the menstrual cycle. It can cause a delayed period or a missed period. When troubles and tensions increase in a PMS sufferer's life, they also take their toll by increasing her symptoms, such as irritability and depression.

Panic can be one symptom of PMS, and the stresses of life as well as the stress of having undiagnosed symptoms only serve to increase the possibility of panic. In fact, professionals who fail to consider this syndrome may misdiagnose the problem as panic disorder. The best way to distinguish the two is for the sufferer to keep a daily chart of symptoms for two or more months. By matching the discomfort with the menstrual cycle, a clear pattern should emerge if you have PMS.

Treatment for PMS must be individualized, since medical science is still exploring the exact causes. Several approaches are considered to have potential benefit. The broadest recommendation is an attention to food, vitamins, exercise, and emotions. Foods to avoid or reduce are highly processed foods, those containing chemicals, and those high in sugar, salt, or fat, and those containing caffeine or alcohol. Controlling eating binges and weight gain can also lower risk. Foods that may be beneficial in reducing symptoms are those high in protein and whole grains, the legume family, seeds and nuts, vegetables, fruits, and foods containing unsaturated vegetable oils. Frequent, smaller meals and a low carbohydrate diet, especially avoiding simple sugars, may be favorable. Calcium supplements (1200–1500 mg/day) have been shown to help. Increased physical exercise promotes an increase in metabolism. And finally, counseling to help in coping with stress is important.

Common prescription medicines for PMS include the SSRI antidepressants, the benzodiazepines, the mild tranquilizer, buspirone, and those that suppress ovulation, such as the GnRH agonists Lupron and Buserelin. The benefits of oral contraceptives are still being researched.

You may find that, even though your symptoms are not identifiable as PMS, they become stronger prior to menstruation. A number of my clients have remarked that they are more likely to panic during this time. Their comments support my belief that hormonal changes can influence susceptibility to anxiety attacks. Specifically, the female hormone progesterone has been found to increase the sensitivity of certain chemical receptors in the body. Progesterone is secreted during the premenstrual phase of a woman's cycle. It is possible then that these alarm systems become too sensitive, causing the brain to respond to misinterpreted signals. This may account in part for the far greater frequency of panic in women than men, as well as the increase in anxiety and irritability during the premenstrual phase.

The symptom of panic in a PMS sufferer can begin to take on a life of its own, causing many complications. In Parts III and IV of this book you will learn to "desensitize" this alarm system so that your symptoms remain under your control. You can manage panic and eventually eliminate it from your life as you find the best treatment for your other PMS symptoms. While some anxiety may persist, no one needs to feel swallowed up by the fear of unexpected, uncontrollable anxiety attacks.

Hypoglycemia

As mentioned in Chapter 2, hypoglycemia (meaning "low blood sugar") is the experience of uncomfortable physical symptoms during times when there is a lower than normal level of glucose in the blood stream. This condition is quite rare and is found predominantly in people with diabetes mellitus. Other causes of "functional" or "reactive" hypoglycemia include high fever, liver disease, pregnancy, stomach surgery, some kinds of cancer, a reaction to certain foods or drugs, and anorexia nervosa.

In diabetes mellitus, the pancreas produces insufficient amounts of insulin, a hormone used to break down and store sugar in the body. One result is a higher than normal amount of glucose in the bloodstream. The disease is managed by means of daily insulin injections and/or a controlled diet. If the diabetic takes too much insulin, does not keep to the prescribed diet, or is engaged in extended strenuous physical activity on a particular day, she may experience a drop in the blood glucose level, leading to symptoms of hypoglycemia.

Severe symptoms of hypoglycemia are indistinguishable from those of a panic attack: trembling, light-headedness, perspiration, anxiety, irritability, tachycardia, unsteadiness, and weakness. The similarity in symptoms is not coincidental. To combat low blood sugar, the medulla of the adrenal glands secretes the hormone epinephrine, which helps release extra sugar from the liver and dump it rapidly into the bloodstream. In addition, epinephrine stimulates the sympathetic branch of the autonomic nervous system. During times of emergency, fear, anger, or threat, epinephrine prepares the body by increasing the heart rate, raising blood pressure, increasing the rate of respiration, tensing muscles, and causing a number of other rapid changes. (This fight-flight-or-freeze response is fully described in Chapter 8.) During a panic attack, the individual believes he is threatened in some way. That belief is enough to signal the brain to cause epinephrine to be secreted.

Since the symptoms of hypoglycemia and panic attacks are so closely related, misdiagnosis is a serious problem. In the past hypoglycemia has been diagnosed by physicians through a five-hour glucose tolerance test preceded by three days of a high-carbohydrate diet. Even such a rigorous evaluation is insufficient, since 25 to 48 percent of normal individuals will experience random periods of low serum glucose levels. An accurate diagnosis requires that the patient experience *symptoms* during those times of low blood sugar and a *relief of symptoms* as the blood sugar rises.

Important information can be obtained by evaluating the patterns of your panic episodes. Ask yourself the following questions:

1. Do I wake up with panic attacks? Blood sugar levels are lowest in the morning, since the body has experienced its longest period of time without a meal. If symptoms occur every morning, not just every few mornings, hypoglycemia might be a factor.

2. Are there regular patterns to my panic attacks? Blood glucose levels are lowest just before lunch, just before dinner, and two to three hours after lunch and dinner. If your panic consistently coincides with one or more of these periods, low blood sugar may be contributing to the problem.

3. Does sugar in some form completely remove the symptoms? If you are prone to panic during these times, experiment with consuming sugar in some form (a sweet roll, fruit juice, candy, or pure sugar) when you begin to panic. If your symptoms consistently diminish within 10 to 30 minutes, you should check with your doctor to consider a diagnosis of hypoglycemia.

A number of popular books have proclaimed hypoglycemia to be the undiagnosed culprit behind a vast number of physical and psychological problems. In fact, the exact opposite may be true. Poor diagnostic procedures by professionals and self-diagnosis by lay people account for the inordinately large number of false cases of hypoglycemia. For instance, in a recent study of 135 patients who claimed to have or were suspected of having hypoglycemia, only 4 could be confirmed with the diagnosis. Eighty percent of the other patients manifested some kind of psychiatric condition, especially depression and somatization, which is the continual focus on multiple physical complaints.

The misdiagnosing of hypoglycemia is a dangerous affair, since a false confirmation of this illness prevents the true diagnosis from being identified and treated. Serious physical problems such as hypertension and hyperthyroidism (described in Chapter 2) may be present, as may treatable psychological problems.

The diagnoses that may be missed are depression, panic disorder, and agoraphobia. There are several reasons for this. First, of course, is the fact that paniclike symptoms can be present in hypoglycemia. There is also a relationship with the times when panic might occur. If a person has a panic attack routinely while standing in line at the grocery store or waiting for a meal in a restaurant, is it panic disorder or hypoglycemia? If the person hasn't eaten in a few hours, she may feel the same jitteriness and other symptoms that any of us might get when our body reacts to a low blood sugar level.

The panic-prone person will not only notice her symptoms while in the store or restaurant, but will react fearfully to them. Unlike the situation with hypoglycemia, consuming some form of sugar to diminish the physical symptoms will not relieve her worry; leaving the scene will.

Many people with panic disorder cling to the belief that they have hypoglycemia instead. This provides them with a number of benefits that all fall under the category of avoidance. Psychological problems continue to carry a stigma for many in our culture. By deciding that they have a physical disorder panic-prone people avoid facing the psychological and stress-related problems in their lives. Hypoglycemia provides relief by placing a clear label on some perplexing and ambiguous symptoms. Treatment of panic disorder also requires dedicated effort on the individual's part. Hypoglycemia offers an easier solution, since the sufferers simply pay special attention to their diets. Some putative hypoglycemia patients not only limit what they eat but begin to restrict their social functioning. This may be a clue that the individual is keeping a firm hold on the label of hypoglycemia as a way to avoid facing more fearful possibilities.

As mentioned earlier, to make the diagnosis of reactive hypoglycemia, the physician must determine that the patient's symptoms are present when the blood sugar levels are at their lowest and are relieved when the blood sugar level rises. Merely performing a glucose tolerance test on patients who experience spontaneous panic attacks is insufficient, since a large minority of normal subjects can show random low glucose levels.

Even when a positive diagnosis of hypoglycemia is made, the panic-prone hypoglycemic person may still have to work at managing her emotional reaction to times of low blood sugar. Here are a few suggestions. Carry sugar in some form with you at all times. When you notice the early signs of an attack, calmly eat some sugar until you begin to feel normal again. Explain to friends how to help you if you become disoriented. Instruct them to give you fruit juice or other sweets until you are able to help yourself. A general maintenance diet for hypoglycemia and any necessary precautions will be explained to you by your physician. Parts II and IV of this book present information that will help you control the physiological reactions of your body during a hypoglycemia attack and remain emotionally calm so that your symptoms can be kept to a minimum.

Depression

It is not surprising that some people who experience anxiety attacks become depressed. When we begin to feel our world closing in on us, when we are unable to face situations that previously caused us no anxiety, when we experience physical symptoms that seem to have no clear cause, self-doubt, discouragement, and sadness are understandable side effects.

Many people who experience panic also complain of symptoms related to depression: a low energy level, feelings of hopelessness, low self-esteem, crying spells, irritability, difficulty concentrating, lack of interest in normal activities, a decrease in sexual desire, difficulty with sleep, and fluctuations in weight.

The relationship between panic disorder and depression has been well established through numerous controlled studies. At the same time, this research indicates that panic disorder, agoraphobia, and depression are distinct problems that happen to coexist within the same individual. A large majority of patients with panic disorder or agoraphobia have had episodes of serious depression. One study found that half the panic disorder and agoraphobia patients entering treatment with a history of depression had experienced at least one major depressive period prior to developing panic disorder or separate from periods of panic. In other words, depression doesn't develop simply in reaction to prolonged struggles with panic but can predate the panic attacks. And your depression can lift, even though a problem with panic may continue.

For the person suffering from panic, the most important issue regarding depression is the way it complicates and slows the recovery process. Consider for a moment the thoughts of an anxious person who experiences panic attacks. She looks to a specific future event and worries, "Can I handle it?" She considers the possibility of failure and says, "It's possible I'll fail." She desires to take some action but says, "I'm too afraid." The panic-prone person wishes actively to engage her world, but is doubtful she can manage specific tasks. As panic lingers in a person's life, her outlook and self-evaluation may take on depressive qualities. The person who is primarily anxious will look to the future with uncertainty. She is not sure how difficult future tasks will be; doesn't know if she will perform up to par or be able to control the situation. She doubtfully questions the future.

If she begins to adopt a more depressed attitude, this uncertainty is transformed into fatalistic expectations. She looks to a specific future event and says, "I won't be able to handle it." She considers the possibility of failure and says, "I'll fail." In the internal struggle between wishing to take action and feeling too afraid, the balance shifts. Instead of doubting the future she becomes more certain of what will happen: "I will not succeed."

An even more self-destructive attitude may arise: "I really don't care that much."

These negative predictions and lack of drive are supported by a pervasive sense of personal worthlessness, as though she is missing the essential traits to be a complete, competent human being. Instead of thinking, "I'm not prepared for *that job*," or "I doubt I can enter *that building*," he begins to think, "I'm inadequate. I don't have what it takes. I don't fit in." As he looks to his past, he finds justification for this feeling. "Things are no different than they've ever been. Nothing has ever made that much difference. My limitations are unchangeable."

Helping someone face panic when he or she has adopted a depressed attitude is a difficult task, for obvious reasons: "If I believe that I am basically inadequate, that nothing ever really changes in my life, that tomorrow will be about the same as yesterday, then why should I bother considering alternatives to my present state of affairs? There seems to be no point."

If you are feeling this kind of depression, you must confront and shift your entrenched attitude to face the challenges presented by panic. Through some means, you must move your attitude from a position of certainty ("Nothing is going to change things") to one of uncertainty. Even an anxious attitude ("I don't know if I can manage this") is an improvement. In fact, this is the position I want and expect my clients to take as they begin facing panic. It is not necessary to embrace some false sense of confidence and assurance, because uncertainty is a major component of adult life. By saying "I'm not sure," you are opening your mind to the possibility of change ("Maybe I won't handle this particular challenge, and maybe I will").

There are two ways to begin changing this depressive attitude. The first is to directly wrestle with your negative beliefs: to listen to how you state those beliefs in your mind, to learn how those statements influence your actions and then to explore other attitudes that might support your goals. The second way is to begin to change your activities even before you change your attitude. Try some specific, small activities, without needing to believe they will help you. Change your patterns of behavior during the day, alter your routine, do some things that you imagine someone else must consider "good for you." There is no requirement that you engage in these new activities with the belief that they will help you. At first, just do them. Don't predict how you are "supposed" to feel during or after them—that will usually be a setup to prove, once again, that "nothing will change." Simply change your patterns as a way of giving yourself experiences that might challenge your beliefs in a small way.

Let me illustrate the purpose of this process by describing its use with another kind of problem. In my practice as a clinical psychologist I specialize in the treatment of anxiety disorders and also in the management of chronic pain syndrome. Years ago I worked as a therapist at the Boston Pain Center, a medical in-patient unit for chronic-pain patients. The facility is designed to help those who have tried every known medical treatment and yet remain in significant physical discomfort because of a physical injury or illness.

The chronic-pain patient and the person suffering from panic disorder share the predominance of depression. Consider the patient who enters the treatment unit with chronic low-back pain. He describes himself as "vegetating in front of the boob-tube all day for the past five years." He perceives himself as useless: he hasn't been able to work in five years and his wife supports the family. He can't even mow the lawn or take out the garbage because of his back pain, much less figure out how to return to productive, paid employment. And "all of the doctors have given up hope" on him, so how could the future be anything else but just like the past or worse?

The in-patient program takes him out of the normal routine of his home and provides a broad range of activities that are designed to challenge this attitude. He lives for four to six weeks among twenty other patients with similar pain problems. He is required to rise first thing in the morning, make his own bed, eat in a group dining room, and attend four support/therapy group meetings a week, plus medical sessions, community meetings, and special outings. To manage his physical pain he attends individual and group physical therapy sessions, receives massages and ice massages, hot packs, ice packs, and whirlpools. He is taught biofeedback and relaxation techniques. His pain medications are slowly diminished and eventually discontinued, as he learns alternative ways to successfully manage his pain.

This is the typical design of a therapeutic community, where the medical staff and patients work together to find the best treatment for each individual. We don't expect every approach to work for every patient. Instead, we provide as many options as possible to discover which combination will be most effective.

But one of the first things that must change is the patient's attitude, since a depressive outlook can prevent any learning. How does that attitude shift? Most frequently it changes because the patient begins to have experiences that don't fit into his negative expectations.

For instance, a low-back-pain patient may complain of an inability to stand or sit for more than twenty or thirty minutes at a time, after which he must lie down to relieve his discomfort. By altering his pattern of activities, the therapeutic community offers him a chance to have new experiences that can change his belief. On day 5 of the program he discovers that he just sat through an hour-and-a-half group therapy session without having to stand or lie down. Then he remembers that this is the third time in two days that he has sat for over an hour. It is this kind of awareness that can lead him to say, "Maybe I can do something to help myself. Maybe things can change."

This is usually the turning point for patients on the Pain Unit. Once they decide that change is possible, they tend to look at any new treatment with a ray of hope. They stop being so certain of failure and begin thinking of their options. Trying each new technique now involves curiosity. "How might I benefit from learning biofeedback?" "I wonder what results I'll get if I do these physical therapy exercises every day for a couple of months?"

If you are suffering from depression, this is the kind of curiosity you must strive for. In Parts III and IV of this book I suggest a number of new techniques and activities for you to practice. You will also learn to directly address your depressive attitude, so you have alternative ways of thinking about yourself and your future. As you proceed, keep in mind the need to confront your negative view. For a while you may have to try the suggestions in spite of thinking, "What's the use?" Above all, you must take action. No matter how low you feel, some part of you believes that you can help yourself. Even if it is a small ember of hope deep within you, let that supportive self give you the gift of curiosity.

Alcoholism

Alcohol can have a dramatic effect on the body. It is primarily a central nervous system depressant, similar to major and minor tranquilizers, barbiturates, narcotics, and nonbarbiturate sleeping pills. It is just as addicting as these drugs in that there is a specific physical and psychological withdrawal process after prolonged use.

As a central nervous system depressant, alcohol slows down the communication among the neurotransmitters in the brain. The first neurotransmitters affected are the inhibitory ones, so alcohol's first effect is usually the removal of tensions and inhibitions. This is the primary reason people with anxiety, fears, or panic might turn to drinking. With alcohol, they typically experience warmth, relaxation, and a general feeling of well-being.

As larger amounts of alcohol are consumed, however, the entire nervous system becomes depressed, leading to impairment in judgment, motor coordination, speech, vision, and balance. And of course, since judgment is distorted, the person drinking in excess is unable to judge the negative behavior changes.

Heavy drinking can lead to a hypoglycemic reaction, usually occurring twelve to sixteen hours after a drinking bout. As the liver metabolizes alcohol, it stops manufacturing glycogen (the precursor to glucose). Blood sugar levels are then maintained by using previously stored glycogen. Once that supply is used up, blood sugar levels drop, producing a hypoglycemic reaction. As mentioned in the earlier discussion of hypoglycemia, this reaction can be indistinguishable from panic. Some panic-prone persons are susceptible to low blood sugar levels. For instance, drinking may diminish their anxiety level during an evening out. Twelve or so hours later, as the next morning begins, they experience panic symptoms that seem to come from nowhere. This of course reinforces their sense of being out of control and may encourage them to take another drink to "calm the nerves."

Several studies have explored alcoholism and phobias, bringing interesting patterns to light. It has been estimated that 5 to 10 percent of all phobic people are dependent on some chemical such as alcohol. Studies of alcoholics indicate a high correlation between the degree of the person's dependence and the presence of phobia.

One study of 102 alcoholics admitted into an alcohol treatment unit in England found that one-third of them also suffered from agoraphobia or a social phobia. Another one-third had phobic symptoms to a less disabling degree. A second study by the same investigators found that in a group of 44 alcoholics who each had a phobia, the majority developed their phobic symptoms prior to their alcohol dependency.

It appears, then, that some panic-prone persons drink to relieve their anxiety and their crutch may end up causing them more serious problems. Often the drinking pattern becomes autonomous: the person still has the same fears and still avoids uncomfortable situations but is now also consumed by alcohol.

I predict that in the years to come, research will continue to confirm this significant relationship: for certain alcoholics, anxieties regarding their abilities to handle themselves in specific situations draw them to drink. For the short term they perceive the drinking to be helping them by diminishing their sense of fear. Yet, as time passes, the alcohol takes on a stronger, independent role in their lives. They increase their alcohol consumption, which actually increases their original problem: their emotional instability and their isolation from family members and friends.

Because of the serious problems caused by alcoholism, phobic symptoms tend to go unnoticed, even within a professional treatment program. Since the symptoms of detoxification are similar to symptoms of anxiety, both the patients and the alcoholism treatment staff may not consider any phobic or panic disorder as an additional diagnosis. When the anxious fears return, though, patients may once again reach for the only relief they know. The more skilled the treatment staff can become in identifying anxiety-related drinking problems, and the more patients can wrestle directly with these issues, the less that revolving door in the detoxification unit will spin.

Dependency on alcohol reinforces a negative belief system. Anxious people can see alcohol as a form of self-medication, but simultaneously their dependency reinforces the belief that they are not in control. They feel safe only after a few drinks. Any difficult situation becomes a cue to reach for a drink. In time, this numbing process replaces self-assurance, confidence, and pride.

As you might imagine, depression in the panic-prone person is another problem that is reinforced by alcohol. The scenario may unfold in dozens of ways. Here is a hypothetical example:

One day, to my great surprise I have an anxiety attack just before making a presentation at a business meeting.

Over the next several weeks I worry about losing control like that again. I'm feeling tense in general these days because of expanded job responsibilities and competition from some others in the company. Before my next presentation I down a shot of whiskey, "just to take the edge off." It actually works: I'm calmer just before my talk and during it. But I continue to remain on edge during the week.

Before a dinner party the next week I again become panicky. Out comes the whiskey to turn the evening into a pleasant time. I am discovering that I can manage the tensions with this little helper, even though I notice an unusual increase in my anxiety level the next morning.

Time passes. It is four months later—four months of swings of tension followed by relief. Four months of doubt about my ability to handle the pressures of work. Four months of distortions in my normal thinking about my job, my life, my capabilities. My anxiety begins to change. Now, instead of thinking, "Oh, no, how will I handle these responsibilities," I begin to think, "I don't really care that much." The persistent drinking to ease the anxiety takes its toll as my anxious feelings become wrapped in a blanket of depressive indifference. "The job's not that important" might be my conscious thought. But underneath this is a growing sense that I am no longer the man I thought I was; I don't have what it takes to control my life, I am stuck and might as well surrender. Nothing will fix the problem, so I can only learn to cope with it.

Through the powerful combination of alcohol and depression, the symptoms of panic have led to a serious and complex syndrome involving denial, self-defeating behaviors, avoidance, loss of self-esteem, and physical deterioration.

If alcohol has become your crutch you must remain alert to its seductiveness. Facing your fears without it may seem tough, but your successes without this drug will provide your only avenue to long-lasting change. If you suspect that you may be dependent on alcohol or if people close to you agree that you have a problem, seek out professional help or the help of self-help organizations such as Alcoholics Anonymous.

CHAPTER 6

Panic in the Context of Heart and Lung Disorders

It is easy to take the human body for granted. Its complex functioning is so phenomenal that we can scarcely imagine the process, much less appreciate it. With nourishment and upkeep, the body runs for decades without any major complaints. All systems work together for one single objective: to maintain equilibrium throughout the body and between the body and its environment.

The cardiovascular and respiratory systems work together as the primary forces behind this process. Through its smooth, rhythmic action, the respiratory system ensures that adequate levels of oxygen are available instantly for any circumstance and maintains the delicate acid-base balance in the blood. The cardiovascular system makes certain that every cell in the body is fed nutrients and oxygen and is cleansed of waste products. The heart circulates five quarts of blood through the body every minute, which also helps the body maintain a constant, comfortable temperature.

Because these two major systems are so vital to our moment-by-moment life, the body and mind will react faster than the speed of light if these systems are threatened. This automatic alarm, evolved over hundreds of thousands of years, directs all our human capabilities with two instructions: "Find any way to breathe, and keep the heart beating."

A dramatic moment eleven years ago still reminds me of this powerful alarm system. I am standing on the porch of my parents' farm in the mountains of North Carolina. My father is holding our twelve-month-old daughter as we talk casually about one thing or another. I glance at Joanna at the same moment her eyes bulge and she stops breathing. I lunge forward and slap her on the back while three other options to free her passageway instantly appear in my mind. Within five seconds from start to finish, the piece of ice that has lodged in her throat has melted and cleared through the esophagus.

As an infant, Joanna hardly knew anything had happened. I, on the other hand, experienced the remarkable speed and skill of my unconscious life-saving instinct. And my body and mind were left with the aftereffects of this psychophysiological response. As soon as I saw that Joanna was breathing again I also noticed that my head was pounding from all the blood that rushed there. And I mean *rushed*. My circulatory system pushed an abundant supply of blood to the vessels of my brain within my first two heartbeats.

This, of course, was only a minor crisis, because no harm was done. But the body doesn't wait around for some panel of experts to vote on the degree of the crisis. If the brain signals "crisis," the body responds. This instinct saves our lives.

People with a chronic heart or lung problem face many new challenges. One of these is how to adjust the signals from the brain so that the minor symptoms of the problem are not interpreted as life-threatening. If patients with heart disease react fearfully to every pressure in their chest, they place unnecessary strain on the healing heart. If patients with emphysema become anxious about every new activity, they directly aggravate their safe, comfortable breathing pattern. And yet, the brain has been trained for hundreds of centuries to shift the body into crisis gear when the heart and lungs seem to be threatened. Therefore, learning to cope with these chronic conditions can be quite challenging.

In disorders of the heart and lungs, panic arises when the body and mind respond to a relatively minor symptom with the weapons typically reserved to combat a life-threatening situation. This chapter discusses five of these conditions: mitral valve prolapse, recovery from myocardial infarction, emphysema, bronchitis, and asthma.

Mitral Valve Prolapse

The mitral valve is a structure within the heart that controls the opening between the left atrium and the left ventricle. In mitral valve prolapse (MVP), this valve leaflet balloons slightly into the left atrium during contractions. (Figure 2 shows the location of the mitral valve and the change in its appearance after ballooning.)

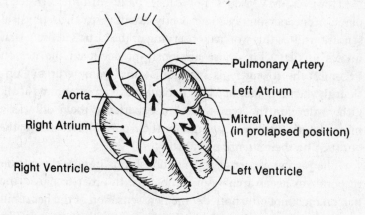

Figure 2. Location of mitral valve and change in appearance after ballooning.

This minor cardiac abnormality is found in approximately 2 percent of all adults. Most people who have this problem are never aware of it, since 50 percent of those with MVP experience no symptoms. On average, even if MVP is identified, no medical treatment is needed. Of the 50 percent who do notice symptoms, the predominant is palpitations, the conscious awareness of some unpleasant sensation of the heart. They may be aware of premature contractions of the heart chambers, (extrasystoles), or of a rapid heartbeat (tachycardia). Other possible symptoms are shortness of breath or difficulty breathing (dyspnea), dizziness, chest pain, fatigue, fainting, and panic attacks. It seems that between 10 and 20 percent of MVP patients experience panic.

Given these symptoms, what is the relationship between panic disorder and mitral valve prolapse? Demographically, they appear to be related. Those with noticeable symptoms of MVP are found with approximately the same frequency as those with panic disorder: approximately 1.5 percent of the population. Both are found more often among women, with symptoms beginning in early adulthood. Research findings indicate that some people with MVP may have inherited it, and so for some individuals there may be a genetic link associating these two problems.

However, MVP does not cause panic disorder. Instead, panic-prone persons become overly attentive to their physical sensations. It is this worried observing of the heart's activity that invites anxiety. The more anxiously preoccupied the person becomes, the stronger his symptoms, until panic erupts. Consider the fact that half of MVP patients have no symptoms at all. Others develop the symptoms but experience them only as a minor nuisance. They continue in their normal activities without turning their attention inward.

The pivotal aspect of this relationship is in how the person responds to his awareness of symptoms. In order to panic, the person must not only notice some new sensation of the heart but must also become fearful of what that sensation means. The autonomic nervous system will then respond to the person's fearful thoughts, not to the heart palpitation itself. This process, fully described in Chapters 7 and 8, produces more dramatic symptoms, such as a racing heart, dizziness, shortness of breath, and even a panic attack.

Since mitral valve prolapse can produce palpitations at random, it contributes to the panic-prone person's commitment to remain "on guard" at all times to defend against mysterious "out-of-the-blue" attacks of panic. One advantage of receiving a clear physical diagnosis of MVP is that it can reassure the panic-prone person that these symptoms are not a sign of danger. By diminishing worry and anxiety you automatically diminish the potential for symptoms.

Diagnosis of mitral valve prolapse is made by a cardiologist through echocardiography, which records the position and motion of the valve by echoes of ultrasonic waves transmitted through the chest wall, and through listening to the sounds of the heart during contraction. Evaluation by a physician is recommended if a person experiences a sudden occurrence of physical symptoms, such as true vertigo (room spinning), fainting, chest pains, or palpitations.

If you are diagnosed with MVP, it's important to understand a few points. First, changes in the rhythm of the heart are a frequent occurrence in most people and are rarely harmful. By learning to accept, tolerate, even ignore them, you will diminish your anxiety. Second, don't let those symptoms frighten you into avoiding activities. By avoiding, you feed a negative pattern that unnecessarily restricts your life. Third, you can actually reduce your symptoms to a few annoying but not distressing sensations by learning to accept the normal process of mitral valve prolapse.

Recovery from Myocardial Infarction

A heart attack is certainly cause for reflection. It is a traumatic blow to the ego which jerks us out of our mundane patterns and calls our attention to the fragility of life. The return to physical health is slow and steady for those with uncomplicated problems, but the psychological recovery almost always includes a struggle with two stresses: depression and anxiety. Depressed patients wrestle with thoughts and feelings of resignation, "My life is no longer worth fighting for."

Anxious patients, on the other hand, feel threatened by the thought, "I might die soon." Their primary question is, "How cautious should I be?" After a heart attack this becomes a complicated question, since its answer affects hundreds of small daily decisions for years to come. It is no wonder that many of these patients continue to restrict their lifestyle and feel uncertain about activities for months and even years beyond the acute phase of the illness. "Will I die at the same age as my father? Should I ever risk having sex again? Will I die in my sleep tonight? I shouldn't be getting excited like this. Is that a pain in my chest as I inhale?"

Post–MI patients can make three basic life-choices:

1. *The healthy stance: Knowing my limits and my options, I work within them to expand them.* There is an old expression that runs, "Freedom is what you do with what's given to you." To experience freedom, post–MI patients who have made this choice work with their physician and other medical professionals to understand their current physical state and capacity. They then learn what activities are possible given this stage in the healing process. They act on their desire to live life to the fullest within those limits, while simultaneously adopting a medical plan that can help expand those limits. This is the only life-choice that will successfully control panic.

2. *The panic-prone stance: I must remain constantly on guard, since the slightest provocation could cause my death.* Panic arises because post–MI patients are unclear about their limits or options. They notice a symptom or potential symptom and have no

specific plan for monitoring or controlling it. This lack of preparation turns their body against them. Without the proper signal of reassurance from the brain, the body reacts by shifting into crisis gear, which causes an increase in symptoms. This life-choice encourages chronic anxiety and panic attacks, which seriously strain the heart.

3. *The depressive stance: There is no point in continuing to try, since my course is now charted.* These patients surrender their power to heal themselves. Because of their willingness to become dependent on others, helpless and restricted in their activities, these patients have been labeled "cardiac invalids." Often they withdraw from friends and retire from work. This life-choice dissolves the spirit to live. By becoming physically passive they worsen their medical status by weakening the cardiovascular and respiratory systems, since regular exercise helps maintain all organs and systems of the body.

The panic-prone stance can lead to the depressive stance, "If I continue to face situations that I believe might stress my heart and do not develop a plan to manage those situations, eventually I must alter my course. My only solution, then, is to avoid those situations." Soon avoidance is the first choice. Since preventing another heart attack is more important than some brief pleasure, they also stop participating in the activities they enjoy. They become less anxious, but lose pleasures too. Depression steps in to fill the void.

If you are recovering from a heart attack, your physician will help you understand your physical limits and will design a rehabilitation course so you can return to your highest level of functioning. Your physician will also help you understand and respond appropriately to any unusual symptoms you might experience.

Parts III and IV of this book offer you information and many skills to use within the context of your medical treatment: how to think clearly in case of any medical emergency, how your attitude toward your health affects your reaction to symptoms, and how to calm yourself if you become anxious or panicky. We know from research and numerous clinical reports that simply mastering a few basic calming skills is one key ingredient to recovery from any cardiovascular illness, including hypertension and coronary artery disease. Most important, you will learn how to return safely to the physical and social activities that give your life meaning and pleasure. Before reading Parts III and IV, discuss with your doctor the appropriate response to various symptoms.

Chronic Obstructive Pulmonary Disease

"I'll never breathe again." That is the statement that screamed out in my mind. And for that instant, I believed it with all my heart, soul, and mind. There was not the tiniest sliver of belief that I would live. You don't live without air. I could not inhale, and I had no air in my lungs at that moment. I was dying. Good-bye.

That moment occurred during the second half of a soccer match a few summers ago. As a defensive fullback, I stepped in front of the offensive forward just as he followed through on a forceful kick toward the goal. The ball slammed into my chest at point-blank range. The power behind the blow knocked all the air from my lungs, leaving me, literally, breathless. The game continued as I stood there, frozen, leaning halfway forward, incapable of inhaling and incapable of speaking. This marked the moment of panic for me: I believed, on the basis of my physical experience, that I did not have the control to save my own life.

My panic lasted about twenty seconds. Within thirty seconds, action had stopped in the match, two teammates had helped me to lie down on the ground, and I had had my first taste of ever-so-precious-but-lost-forever air.

I can look back now and laugh a bit at my extreme reaction to such a benign occurrence. On the other hand, this was the second time in three months that I had lost my breath on the playing field. And during both moments I thought, "I'll never breathe again." The panic associated with heart or lung problems is special. You don't experience it as a passing moment, you experience it as your *last* moment.

Panic plays its most damaging role in patients suffering from chronic obstructive pulmonary disease (COPD). The illnesses interfere with the natural breathing process and diminish vitality and endurance. For some patients, the symptoms become more severe over the years. If the illness progresses, they become less and less able to work or to enjoy social and recreational activities, since any kind of exertion or emotional shift could trigger a breathing problem. Anxious patients with a chronic lung problem learn to brace themselves for any sign of discomfort and often choose to avoid activities to feel safe. This is the fearful stance, which is most vulnerable to panic.

The essential feature in many respiratory disorders is a narrowing of the bronchial tubes. In chronic bronchitis, the mucous membrane that lines the main air passages, or bronchi, of the lungs becomes inflamed. This leads to breathlessness, coughing that brings up phlegm, and an increased risk of infection. In chronic asthma, the muscles of the bronchial walls contract, causing a partial obstruction of the bronchi and the bronchioles, the smaller air passages in the lungs. The patient experiences attacks of wheezing and has difficulty breathing, triggered by allergy-provoking substances, physical activity, or psychological stress. With chronic emphysema, the air sacs, or alveoli, at the ends of the bronchioles are damaged. Since these are the site of oxygen and carbon dioxide exchange, the lungs become less and less efficient at their job. The primary symptom is difficulty breathing, which worsens over the years. Figure 3 identifies the parts of the respiratory system affected by these diseases.

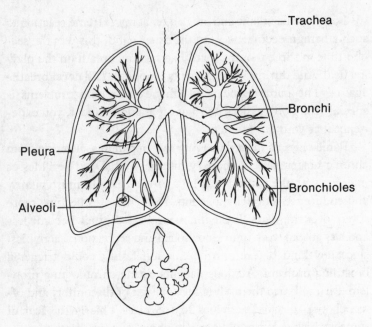

Figure 3. Parts of respiratory system affected by chronic obstructive pulmonary disease.

Since breathing is one of the two most prominent life-supporting processes (along with the pumping of your heart), patients with COPD are likely to develop anxiety, panic, and depression because of their inability to control this vital function. Their most-feared problem is having difficulty breathing. When an episode of difficult breathing begins, they may respond with panic, believing that they will die from suffocation as they gasp for breath. This brief period of panic becomes etched in their mind. The aftereffects of this trauma are maintained by vivid recollections of the attack, by nightmares of being unable to inhale, and by thoughts that the next attack could come anytime, anywhere. The results of one study illustrate the outcome of such recurring experiences: The researchers found that 96 percent of the subjects with COPD developed "disabling" anxiety.

As they withdraw from their world to protect themselves from anything that might cause breathlessness, the patients' general level of anxiety may diminish. But they then become susceptible to depression. If people are socially isolated, cut themselves off from pleasurable activities, and avoid conflicts, strong emotions, or any new experiences, they set themselves up to become a victim of depression.

Dr. Donald Dudley of the University of Washington aptly states that many severely disabled COPD patients live in "emotional straightjackets." It is no wonder, since any shift in emotion, whether toward anxiety, joy, or depression, can trigger a physiological reaction. This impending sense of doom can translate into obsessions, compulsions, phobias, and ritualistic behaviors. Some will even become fearful of visits to their physicians. Depression, fueled by low self-esteem and hopelessness, can lower patients' motivation to participate in important treatment programs.

I want to emphasize the degree to which emotions have a direct mechanical effect on the respiratory system. Since COPD patients have limited pulmonary reserves, their ability to supply oxygen throughout the body and remove carbon dioxide is compromised. Each emotional state has a corresponding breathing pattern. For most people these changes are easily accommodated. However, patients with a severe COPD problem become incapable of managing even minimal changes in respiration.

For example, as we become angry, afraid, or anxious, these more active emotional responses require an increase in metabolism. This need for metabolism cues the respiratory system to increase breathing, to increase the oxygen supply and remove excess carbon dioxide. COPD patients may be physically incapable of accomplishing this increase in breathing. Instead of taking in more air, they begin to have difficulty taking in enough air. The oxygen level in their bodies drops as the amount of carbon dioxide increases. As the difficulty persists, of course they become anxious, causing more symptoms, in a vicious circle of symptoms producing anxiety producing symptoms.

A similar process can take place if patients experience episodes of sadness, depression, or apathy. These emotional states lower the rate of respiration, which leads to low levels of oxygen and high levels of carbon dioxide in the body.

Even if COPD patients are able to inhale sufficiently, they may still become anxiously aware of the increased demand placed on their lungs by an emotional state. In normal circumstances the breathing pattern matches the demands placed on the body. When I am involved in a vigorous physical activity, the increased oxygen my lungs supply is utilized efficiently during metabolism. During anxious moments, however, the body often cannot use the oxygen as rapidly as it is put into the bloodstream. At the same time, the lungs remove more carbon dioxide from the body than is useful. The result is hyperventilation, which causes a number of uncomfortable symptoms in addition to those caused by the illness. A complete overview of breathing processes and hyperventilation is presented in Chapter 16.

If you suffer from a serious COPD, managing your daily living presents a great challenge. Often your predicament seems hopeless. But you can bring a beneficial attitude and set of skills to this challenge. I believe that those suffering the discomforts of COPD can begin to feel safe and more involved in their life and community by considering the suggestions and practicing the skills described in this book. Here are several guidelines which may help you along the way as you read Parts III and IV:

1. Your central goal should be to find as many ways as possible to keep physically active and maintain your interest in life without harming yourself. Setting realistic goals and working progressively and safely toward them will improve your spirits, strengthen your respiratory system, and decrease any unrealistic fears you may have.

2. When you socialize, find ways to make yourself comfortable. Some people become easily fatigued and must end an evening earlier than expected. Those with chronic bronchitis may have to tolerate a severe coughing spell and dispose of sputum discreetly. To remain active you will need to find ways to handle these situations without withdrawing in embarrassment.

3. If you are taking medications, discuss with your physician whether any of them might cause increased nervousness or irritability. For instance, certain drugs help open up the bronchi by activating the sympathetic nervous system, which may make you feel a little more jumpy. Knowing this can help you prepare for any mild side effects. Three classes of medication used for COPD patients are the medications most likely to cause unpleasant side effects. The oral medications used for bronchospasm—aminophylline and the beta-Z adrenergic agents—can cause general anxiety and a rapid heartbeat. People who use an inhaler of the beta-Z adrenergic agents such as isoproterenol and metaproterenol can experience general anxiety and shaky hands. The corticosteroids, such as Prednisone, may briefly elevate the patient's mood, then cause a swing into depressed feelings.

4. The problems of your life will not disappear just because you avoid them. Your best approach is to learn ways of facing and coping with any stressful changes. If you don't respond to the curves that life throws you, then you will eventually surrender control of your life.

5. If you suffer from a severe lung disease, you may find it necessary to avoid any situation that causes anxiety or can lead to any rapid change in your emotional state. It is sometimes a tricky balancing act to remain an interested participant in your world and at the same time not become too caught up in the dramas of life.

6. When nervousness, worry, and depression do come, learn how to diminish them by applying skills such as those described in Parts III and IV. The less worried you are, the fewer severe breathing episodes you will have and the less you will need to use emergency care.

Most important, learn the best ways to think, feel, and act during an acute episode of difficult breathing. You can learn specific techniques that minimize symptoms and support your return to comfortable breathing. The breathing problems that confront COPD patients are quite unique. Our bodies and minds do not instinctively respond to these attacks in a supportive way. In fact, it appears that some of our instinctive reactions cause symptoms to get worse. It is necessary, therefore, to study your individual patterns and adjust them to diminish your anxiety and increase your sense of well-being. You must develop the ability to notice your symptoms without reacting emotionally to them. By learning a set of response skills, by creating a plan for when and how to use them, and then by repeatedly practicing them, you will begin to take control of the symptoms of your illness. Anyone would react with anxiety to the thought of not being able to breathe. Your task is to reduce your anxiety once you notice it and then take steps to improve your breathing pattern.

The Nature of

PART II

Anxiety Attacks

CHAPTER 7

The Anatomy of Panic

The battleground of panic is not isolated to the few seconds or few minutes of an anxiety attack. The more panic attacks you experience without gaining mastery over them, the more they seem to invade other territories. Imagine for a moment that panic is an enemy that has chosen to wrest control of your life away from you. The cleverest of invaders will overcome their victims by undermining their foundations, withholding their nourishment, destroying their confidence. And that's just what panic will do, given the chance.

The first panic attack can be a surprise, to be dismissed as a fluke. Two panic attacks might be viewed as coincidence; you rationalize that too much stress caused the problem. You tell yourself to slow down, take it easy, don't get uptight. However, if the episodes continue, panic makes its first inroads into your life. You begin to question yourself, to doubt your strength, to wonder whether you are coping. This is panic's most powerful weapon. This is what begins to loosen the bricks in your foundation. By creating self-doubt, panic gains its first stronghold in your life. After a while, the panic attack itself plays a role in the ongoing battle. With all the cleverness of a magician, panic appears in your life; and with all the swiftness and power of a judo master, panic takes your mental energy and turns it against you. Before you know it, you've reversed the tables on yourself. Just as with any of the martial arts, the more you fight panic, the more you seem to lose.

Am I overstating the case? I don't think so. People who call my office for a first appointment usually have experienced panic attacks for anywhere from six months to dozens of years. Here are some of the many ways panic, over a period of time, can use your thoughts, feelings, and beliefs as weapons against you:

- Some reminder causes you to hesitate before venturing back into the arena of that last attack.
- The need to avoid becoming "trapped" is given high priority each time you consider certain activities.
- You anxiously wonder when the next attack will come. "Will it be here, now?" Simply asking the question seems to bring on anxiety.
- You nervously think about the last panic attack, and then you doubt your control over your body.
- You worry that some unknown physical illness or an emotional breakdown is causing your attacks.
- If you have a diagnosed physical illness, you fear any undue stress or aggravation.
- You begin to avoid certain people or places as your principal defense against attack.
- You become more socially isolated and secretive, perhaps feeling trapped by appointments, roles, expectations.
- You brood, you worry, you criticize yourself and become discouraged.
- You may stop trusting yourself and turn to alcohol, drugs, or doctors to carry you through your days.

You can see that portraying the anatomy of panic requires a broader brush than you might at first imagine. Every individual is unique, and the ways panic affects each of us are different. There are no absolutes, this is not a black-and-white picture of straight lines and curves. There are many gray areas and a number of frightening shadows. For each person the intensity, duration, and depth of the specific problem areas differ. To help yourself you must first paint an accurate picture of your unique situation. Only then can you decide how you must change that picture to regain control. I describe many serious problems encountered by my clients, but in no way do I mean to suggest that you will face these same difficulties. Please read these passages with a curious mind, asking yourself whether that particular aspect relates to your experience. For example, the inability to understand why you are experiencing an anxiety attack can dramatically increase your anxiety. I address this problem and ways to handle it in a number of sections of this book. On the other hand, readers who suffer from chronic bronchitis, emphysema, or asthma *know* why they panic—they become afraid that they won't be able to get enough air. These readers will not need to focus on this "why" issue.

The first change you achieve will probably be a greater understanding of how panic affects you as an individual. But knowledge alone will never be enough. You must then evaluate your way of thinking about yourself and the world you have created around you, your beliefs about yourself and your roles, your emotions, especially the feelings you are afraid of, and your actions—the things you do and don't do. Panic invades all four arenas, so you must gain control of each territory to regain control of your life. The keys to long-lasting change are challenging your attitude about your present-day life, exploring the roots of your many beliefs, learning from your emotional responses, and experimenting with new actions.

One of your strongest resources for overcoming panic is knowledge, since panic uses doubt, uncertainty, and fear of the unknown as its powerful allies. At this point you should know whether your problem with panic is serious enough to merit a diagnostic evaluation by a physician or a mental-health professional. If a physical or psychological disorder is diagnosed, learn as much as you can about it: What is its cause? What are the other problems associated with it? What professional help will you need? How can you help yourself? A broad understanding of your situation will serve as the foundation of your success.

This book is designed to address all the issues central to panic attacks. Let's begin by separating panic into its component parts. How does it disrupt your confidence? In what ways does it make you a victim of its surprise attacks?

The central element of panic, of course, is its uncomfortable sensations, which I described in Chapter 1. Needless to say, if this book is going to help you, it must advise you on how to manage that discomfort. In Chapter 8 you will learn about the physiology of panic, and in later chapters you will gain the tools necessary to become master of your body again. Now, however, I want you to think about the ways brief episodes of anxiety can play havoc by disrupting your thoughts.

Winning Through Intimidation

The only way panic gains control over you is through psychological intimidation. The actual panic attacks last only an infinitesimal amount of time. Even if you had one panic episode every day and that episode lasted five minutes, you would be experiencing panic only one-third of a percent of your life—and yet some people can become completely dominated by the repercussions of those moments of panic.

Consider the concept of "losing control." What does that mean to you? For most people it means losing security, safety, protection. If we have a sense that we are out of control, we immediately, almost instinctively, begin searching for some small way to regain our equilibrium, whether we have lost control of that burst water pipe in the basement, or slippery roads have caused a momentary loss of steering, or our young child has disappeared from sight in a shopping mall.

And after you have lost control once, what do you do? You probably start checking *all* the pipes in the basement to make sure there aren't any more potential breaks. A few hours later you might go back down those stairs "just to check and see if everything's OK" After momentarily losing control on the highway you may grip the steering wheel a little tighter, even chastise yourself for being overconfident and driving with one hand. Once you find your missing child in the mall you probably begin a constant vigil over her whereabouts. *When the mind fears loss of control, it thinks more intensely about how to keep control in the future.*

Panic attacks—especially spontaneous attacks—stimulate the sense of being out of control. All of a sudden you are not in charge of your body. Heart, lungs, throat, head, legs—all seem to have minds of their own. That is very frightening. Just the thought of it can make you anxious.

And that is how it begins, how panic starts to invade your life. You fear that those uncomfortable physical sensations might return yet again. And how bad will they get? Worse than before? You don't know. It is not knowing that proves to be a devastating weapon: "Since I didn't manage the last attack, how can I possibly handle this one?"

The Surprise Attack

To add to your confusion, the attacks are not always consistent. You might get hit with anxiety at a restaurant one evening, have a problem only once over the next three times you go out for dinner, then on your fifth time out begin to feel the same trapped sensation again. It is like spinning the chamber of the pistol in Russian roulette. Mentally, and even physically, you brace yourself in anticipation. You become constantly on guard. For some, these fears translate into a desperate need not to feel trapped, because being trapped implies surrendering control. "Staying in control" is the primary objective.

Katherine M. is a twenty-nine-year-old single woman who works as an editor for a computer software company. She had been experiencing anxiety attacks for about nine months when I first saw her. Her first moment of panic occurred completely un-expectedly as she was walking to work from the subway station. But as is often the case, this morning was preceded by several months of stress: her boyfriend had broken off their relationship, her boss had been transferred, a close friend had been diagnosed with a terminal illness, and Katherine was seriously considering moving from her hometown of Philadelphia to California.During the past nine months since the first panic attack, her fears and her self-imposed limits have gradually restricted Katherine's world.

Here is how she described some of her concerns when I first interviewed her: "I work downtown, but I won't walk around out-side when I'm there. I'm afraid I'm going to pass out. If I went out to lunch I would be afraid I wouldn't make it back. I also have trouble driving. I get afraid I'll be trapped if I get into the outside lane or if I'm not near an exit. Restaurants bother me. Again it's that trapped feeling: once the order is taken, I can't leave."

Katherine and millions like her suffer from panic disorder. They experience unexpected anxiety attacks and seek a safe asylum from that sense of being trapped. Before venturing out of their place of security they mentally evaluate each new envi-ronment. If they can imagine any chance of being trapped, they avoid the situation. When such avoidance behavior dominates their lives, the diagnosis of agoraphobia is considered.

The fears are not only of being trapped, but of any experi-ence that might produce a sense of being out of control. In Chapter 4 you were introduced to Ann C., a thirty-nine-year-old woman who has experienced agoraphobia for twelve years. Listen to her concern in this brief anecdote.

ANN: When I had surgery for a biopsy, they were going to put me to sleep. The scariest part of the ordeal to me was being put to sleep. I asked the doctor to give me a local anesthetic instead of a general. He said, "You know, you're so brave. Many people say, 'Knock me out, knock me out.'" I said to myself, "Little does he know that my fear *is* of being knocked out, of just *letting go.*"

Why does Ann fear general anesthesia? Because she believes that the way to remain in control of her life is always to be on guard, to monitor her every action, always to watch for potential threats. This belief is actually causing her psychological and physiological discomfort. The mind and body will react to the pressure of constantly bracing for an emergency. It is no wonder that she also reports feeling tense, anxious, and physically and emotionally exhausted.

Panic plays on the imagination. It gains its greatest power through the thoughts and images that you create in your mind. A person who fears elevators doesn't get anxious only while standing in front of an elevator. When he thinks of calling his physician for an appointment, he remembers that the doctor's office is on the fifteenth floor. He reminds himself immediately of his fear. And now, weeks before the appointment, he feels afraid. While sitting in his living room he imagines himself standing in front of the elevator. Then he begins to feel a little light-headed, and he changes his mind about calling his doctor. Most likely he will rationalize his decision, attributing it to more than just fear ("I don't *need* an appointment, yet. I'll just wait a while").

Dorothy P. is another agoraphobic whom I described in Chapter 4. In the following comments, notice how she anticipates losing control. She imagines the worst possible scenario, and this mental image scares her from driving.

DOROTHY: I don't want to lose my license, so I just don't drive. If I had a panic situation driving somewhere—if there was a detour or if traffic backed up—I'd either have to get out and run or jam on the brakes, knock everybody down, knock the policeman down, go through red lights. . . . I would have to escape. I can't seem to say, "Well now, calm down. You know you can. It's only going to be a short time." I can't rationalize it, I don't think at all.

Dorothy is right: she *doesn't* think rationally about her driving skills. The fact is that she has never had an auto accident and has never responded with such hysteria while driving. But she imagines the *possibility,* and that image is enough to keep her out of the driver's seat.

Controlling the Mind

Panic controls more in its victims than just those brief moments of physical anxiety. It connects physical sensations directly with your thoughts, so that simply by entertaining an idea, you stimulate a physical reaction.For example, the *thought* of biting into a lemon can cause the lips to purse. The *thought* of a violent crime can make the muscles tense with anger or fear. The *thought* of sinking into a bath . . . a nice long, deep, warm, soothing, quiet, peacefully restful bath . . . can begin to relax those same tense muscles.

With panic, the body responds to the mind in a similar fashion. I asked Katherine what happens after she has ordered in a restaurant and then thinks of being trapped. "I get terribly anxious and panicky. I'll sit there and eat, so no one will notice. But I become very uncomfortable physically, even dizzy. It's the same when I stand in line at the bank. Once I get to the teller's window and hand my business through, I get very nervous. Because I think, 'I can't leave until she gives me my receipt. I'm stuck!' I start thinking that I'm going to pass out." Katherine remains under control while she is in line only because she tells herself, "I can just get out of the line and leave." But once she begins her transaction, she imagines that she cannot leave without "causing a scene."

Another client, Michelle R., a regional manager of a national corporation, had been experiencing panic episodes for six years.

Her first spontaneous panic was while driving her car. She became dizzy and light-headed and felt as if she was going to faint. After her second attack four months later, she visited her family physician, who diagnosed the problem as "nerves." During the months prior to the onset of her anxiety, Michelle became involved in an extramarital relationship. Within one month, she and her husband separated. Even with the episodes of panic and her physician's diagnosis, Michelle remained calm and unemotional regarding her relationship troubles and saw no connection between her discomfort and her marital conflict. During those next six years she managed her panic disorder without any professional help. She divorced her husband and two years later married the man with whom she had become involved.

By the time of her first appointment with me, she had stopped driving. She never took a walk, or stayed home alone, or shopped alone. In her business she continually found excuses to avoid out-of-town meetings. In addition, I suspected that she was subtly sabotaging her chances for further promotion.

In one of our sessions Michelle described how she gained some insight into the ways panic plays havoc with the mind. During her previous appointment I had asked her to listen for the silent statements she makes just prior to a panic episode. She entered this session with a satisfied smile on her face and said: "Now I know what you mean. I produced my own anxiety attack! I was sitting at a staff meeting this morning and I did it to myself without knowing it. I thought, 'What happens if you feel overwhelmed, or you get that panicky feeling?' And I started feeling it! I could sense my heart racing. I became intensely nervous."

Michelle had always described her panic attacks as coming out of nowhere. In fact, that was one of the worst parts of her experience: she never had a clue as to when or why they would appear. Once she learned that particular ways of thinking can influence physical sensations, she started paying attention to some of her thoughts. In this way she was able to discover one typical line of patter. She would simply mentally raise the possibility of experiencing sensations; then the discomfort seemed to begin. In the past she had not been aware of these thoughts going on in her mind, so the only thing she noticed was her physical reaction. As soon as she discovered she could produce physical discomfort by the way she was thinking, she improved rapidly. She realized that if thoughts could bring on panic, controlling thoughts could also get rid of panic.

Forecasting the Future

Sheryll W., whom you met in Chapter 4, became agoraphobic after the birth of her oldest child twenty-two years ago. She began to feel uncomfortable in church and in grocery stores. Then the anxiety attacks started. "When I panic, my heart rate increases, I hyperventilate, feel dizzy, my legs get weak, especially if I'm experiencing a lot of stress. If I even *think* about going to the beach or another crowded place, I get that smothering feeling and I can't catch my breath. That brings on all the other feelings." Her comments illustrate the same process that Katherine and Michelle describe. As soon as they begin to think negatively about the future, they fall into the panic trap.

It is as though panic has implanted a small voice in your mind. Let's say that you have had some anxious feelings about driving long distances on the highway. Today you decide to drive to your sister's house, fifteen miles away. As the time to leave approaches, that little voice begins. "Now, can you get there without having an anxiety attack? Really and truly get all the way there?" That's all it needs to say, because that question alone plants a seed of doubt in your mind. "Are you a hundred percent certain you can get there? And what if you start to panic . . . then what?" These kinds of questions imply that you *can't* get there without being anxious and that you can't handle the anxiety.

How does panic reach the body through the mind? First, you contemplate venturing into a type of situation that has caused problems in the past. ("I think I'll go grocery shopping today.") Second, you remind yourself that this situation has the *potential* to stimulate your physical sensations. ("Oh, no, last week when I went with the kids I got so dizzy I thought I'd pass out.") Third, you doubt your ability to handle those sensations. ("Who knows what would happen if I went alone? I'd be so humiliated if I had to run out of there. I'm already feeling queasy just thinking about it.")

Your fears may be completely irrational. A part of you may even say, "I know I'll be fine. I've never fainted. Even if I do faint, I'll survive." But despite that voice of logic, the fearful doubts remain. You gradually become plagued by the *concept* of losing control, and that plaguing fear seems to defy logic.

You can now see what a powerful ally panic has if it can instill in your mind a fear of losing control. Add to that fear the uncertainty about when the anxiety will hit and how long the attack will last, and you can see why so many who suffer from panic become physically and emotionally exhausted. They force themselves to be on twenty-four-hour sentry duty!

The Planned Retreat

Only one defensive move seems to bring relief from panic: avoidance. "If I can just keep from having to give that speech [take an airplane, confront my boss, use an elevator], then I'll be fine." And so you retreat to some safe ground. Remaining safe becomes your highest priority.

For certain fears, avoidance can be an acceptable solution. City dwellers needn't be comfortable confronting snakes. Nor does everyone have to be comfortable crossing suspension bridges. But for too many people, avoidance has a significant impact on the quality of their lives. I have worked with clients who have given up driving, who have stopped entering stores or taking buses, who have refused promotions or quit work altogether, who haven't been in a restaurant or to a party in years. I have had to visit some agoraphobics in their homes because they refused to venture outside.

In reaction to an actual physical illness some people will dramatically alter their lives. For instance, I worked with a twenty-four-year-old woman who had suffered from asthma since she was twelve. As you probably know, the symptoms of an asthma attack include wheezing, tightness in the chest, and difficulty breathing. Even though she had not had an asthma attack in over a year, Joella was profoundly fearful of having a spontaneous attack. She rarely traveled beyond her hometown. When she did drive outside the city limits, she would mark on her map the location of each hospital along her route. She would not venture a route unless she thought she could reach a hospital emergency room for oxygen within five minutes. In addition, she remained afraid of ever becoming "too excited," which might trigger a bout of asthma.

Dorothy P. had not traveled outside a two-mile radius of her house in over forty years, nor had she ever been alone during that time.

I don't actually go someplace and panic, because I just tell myself I can't go. I never leave Chapel Hill. Anytime I travel in Chapel Hill I have someone with me. If I go into a restaurant I have to watch the door, even sit near the door. I very seldom go to the movies, and when I do go I take the aisle seat. I have to walk out to the lobby from time to time, and I always leave before the end of the show.

I hate to say this, but I haven't had any anxiety symptoms in years, because I never push myself. I stay away from all things that might produce this trapped feeling.

Few people go to such extreme measures to protect themselves, but many people hesitate in their everyday life. They delude themselves about what they want and need out of life. Actually, they begin talking in terms of what they *don't* want or need: "I don't really want to get all dressed up tonight. Why don't we skip that party? Who needs the added pressure of that promotion? I'd love to meet with you next week, but I don't want to make commitments so far in advance. I never know what might come up."

Some cardiac patients, frightened of overexertion or overexcitement, can become socially isolated and physically inactive. Their fear of triggering a heart attack becomes masked behind indifference and depression. "I'm too old to start taking walks around the block" really means, "What if that walk is all that it takes to produce another attack? I don't want to die." Such fear is understandable, but when it takes primary control over most of your daily activities, you are being run by panic.

Sam S. was a sixty-three-year-old plumber referred to me by his family physician. He had developed the common signs of agoraphobia: he was afraid to ride the subway, take a bus, or drive. He remained home most of the time. And he had developed a peculiar fear of his plumber's tools, which prevented him from returning to work.

After our first interview I had a strong sense that I understood the cause of his problems. After four sessions, my hunch was confirmed. With my encouragement and a few simple suggestions, Sam was able again to take the subway and drive his own car. But his tool phobia was immovable. He said his fears were so great that he couldn't consider the idea of touching the tools without feeling tense and anxious. In fact, he said his fears were so great that he didn't wish to continue treatment. I never saw him again, but I learned from his physician that six months later he still remained out of work.

What did I believe was behind Sam's phobia? Three months before he first saw me, Sam had had his second heart attack. This brush with death triggered his fears of travel and activity. But most important, he feared causing his own death by bringing on a third heart attack. Sam had unconsciously found a way to prolong his life. By developing a phobia toward his tools, he would not have to pick them up again. He would no longer have to crawl under a person's house, lift a twenty-two-pound plumber's wrench, strain to tighten down a joint, and place his weakened heart under that kind of stress.

At his age and after two heart attacks, perhaps Sam *should* have considered retiring his tools. But panic took that decision away from him. He did not consciously feel that he had any choice in the matter. Even explaining my sense of the problem to him had no effect. Panic won, and last I heard, Sam was applying for one-hundred percent disability because of his phobia.

This case illustrates how panic can disrupt the healing process after a physical illness. Regardless of what produces the initial worries or anxieties—whether the cause is emotional or physical—panic can take on an identity of its own and continue to play havoc with a person's life.

Why Me?

If you suffer from unexpected panic attacks that defy all methods of self-control, you want desperately to know *why*. Typically you discover one or both of the following: there is something physically wrong with you or you are experiencing some psychological trouble.

If you remain convinced that the problem is physical despite objective findings to the contrary, you will begin a long and frustrating pilgrimage from doctor to doctor. You might take that same route if you consider the problem to be psychological. Or you may feel so humiliated by the possibility of being labeled "mentally disturbed" that you hide behind the cloak of secrecy. Some of my clients have never told a single person about their years of silent anxiety. Adding to the pain of social isolation is the destructive force of self-doubt and criticism. You blame yourself for your "weakness": "Why am I so afraid? Why don't I just *do it*?"

Panic attacks that defy simple cures can lead a person into a self-destructive downward spiral. Since you feel that you cannot control your life, you gravitate toward any person or thing that might provide that control for you. Through your physician you may try tranquilizers, sedatives, muscle relaxants, or antidepressants. Or you may begin to self-medicate, using alcohol to "take the edge off." Some adults unconsciously choose to remain very close to their parents, even though consciously they feel ambivalent about that decision. Others gravitate toward strong and dominant friends or unconsciously choose a spouse who is powerful and controlling, as a means of feeling safe. These choices are the result of a belief system that follows the line, "Since I know that I am inadequate, I must find someone who will stay close to me and watch over me."

Panic begins to erode your self-confidence by convincing you that you are no longer in control of your life. After a few months, you may face a new set of problems: a loss of drive, diminished motivation, a sense of hopelessness, helplessness, worthlessness. Not only are you feeling out of control of your body, but the people around you seem to be taking control of your life decisions. In other words, panic gains further inroads in your life by its ability to elude cure. It becomes the great unsolvable mystery. You surrender to your panic and loss of control while watching desperately for something or someone powerful enough to conquer it.

The following paragraphs are excerpts from therapy sessions with four of my clients whom you met in Chapter 4. I have taken these passages out of context, so of course a great deal of information is missing. Nonetheless, read between the lines to imagine how such experiences of helplessness can erode the self-confidence and hope of these women.

ANN: After my honeymoon I returned to work and felt utter tension all the time, with very bad headaches and several anxiety attacks. I finally visited the psychiatrist. He put me on Valium [a mild tranquilizer]. I would go to see him each week, but I never got anywhere because he never did any talking. In the end I said, "What's wrong with me? Just what is wrong?" And he said, "Well, you suffer from classic, classic tension." That was his answer.

DONNA: The doctor put me in the hospital for four weeks. During the first week I had all kinds of physical tests, and then I went over to the psychiatric unit for observation for three weeks. That cost us nearly fifteen thousand dollars. And when they were through, they said to me, "We don't know what's wrong with you." The psychiatrist said, "You're as sane as I am," and the medical doctor said, "We can't find anything physically wrong with you." I've tried Valium, Stelazine, Tofranil, and Elavil. They had absolutely no effect. So the doctors said to me, "We're taking you off of all medication and we're discontinuing your psychiatric treatment because there's nothing we can do for you."

KAREN: When I had my second child, I finally was diagnosed as having "cabin fever." I tried to understand it and tried to rationalize it, saying, "Well, you've got two little babies under the age of two, and you have cabin fever. It's the middle of February, and it's a terrible time for people." But deep inside I knew it was something more than that.

SHERYLL: The symptoms began after Susan was born, my oldest. I had postpartum depression, but I also kept experiencing anxiety attacks. One afternoon I was on the phone trying to find an apartment. I started to have chest pains and other symptoms. I called my mother, and they rushed me to the doctor's. They thought I was having a heart attack. That's how it all started. I found that when I went to church I would have a problem. Before long, it was supermarkets. And then I think it all mushroomed. I went to doctor after doctor, and they all said it was my nerves.

As you can see, the mystery that surrounds panic also feeds the panic. To label anxiety attacks as "nerves" and to offer only medications rarely succeeds. In fact, when those medications fail to eliminate panic attacks, the sufferers will often become more distressed. Some people are very secretive. Here is how Katherine described her feelings:

KATHERINE: I think I was just ashamed. I thought I was having a nervous breakdown. I mean, I couldn't just go up to my friends and say, "Hi. I'm having a nervous breakdown." I guess I didn't know how to talk to anyone about it. I thought they would laugh at me. Besides, I don't like to bother people with my problems. People have their own problems, they don't need mine. Or they won't take me seriously. They'll say, "Don't worry about it."

So instead of giving her friends a chance to support her and express their care, Katherine became more withdrawn and turned to alcohol for control.

KATHERINE: I didn't know what was happening to me. And I was also drinking a lot. I would get home at night and drink to calm myself down. There were some weeks when I'd go home and drink half a pint of whiskey at night. I didn't understand what was happening to me, and it seemed to be the only thing that would calm me down. But the alcohol didn't work, because the next day I would feel terrible and the symptoms seemed to be worse.

What accounts for such dramatic physiological changes that defy simple cures? How does panic remain so powerful, yet so mysterious? Part of the answer, discussed in Chapter 8, lies in our inability to trust our bodies' unconscious control. And another part of the answer, examined in Chapter 9, lies in the way we think during times of crises.

Who's in Control?

To me, there is little that brings such peace and serenity as a walk along the beach during the quiet of the early morning. It's as though it's just me and the universe having our private time together, undisturbed. The problems of home seem so far away as I let my mind just drift in its own easy thoughts. The sun slides up over the Atlantic; it looks so big and orange. Everything seems wondrous: the sand crabs digging deeper, leaving only a small hole for the next wave to wash over; the school of dolphins in the near distance diving one way, then the next, through the surface of their playground; the seagulls seeming to hang carelessly in the sky. The ocean shore changes my perspective and slows my busy thoughts. Life seems simpler. The natural world surrounding me invites me to join in its rhythm.

There appears to be a balance in this universe of ours, which is maintained by constant change. The tides of the sea are either in the process of rising or in the process of falling. Nothing is still. Everything in nature is in constant flux, but it is not random change. Just as the pendulum swings, the rhythms of this world seem to produce a balance between two poles. Every molecule in the universe expands and contracts.

Our years on earth are balanced between the heat of summer and the cold of winter. Our days move from the brightness of noon to the darkness of midnight. The rhythm of living things brings movement between rest and activity. For many of us, every twenty-four hours bring sixteen hours of activity and eight of rest. We work five days and rest two days. Each year we balance months of work with weeks of play.

This rhythm is equally profound in the human body. Consider the heart. It expresses a singular pattern as it beats within the chest: contract, relax, contract, relax, contract, relax. Blood doesn't flow through the body; it pulses. Push, relax, push, relax. Each blood vessel expands and contracts as needed, rhythmically.

When you receive a blood pressure reading, you are given two numbers. The higher number—the systolic pressure— indicates the greatest force exerted by the heart and the highest degree of resistance put forth by the walls of your arteries as blood is pumped. The lower number—the diastolic pressure—identifies the lowest pressure in the arteries, at the time when the heart is most relaxed. Your pulse rate expresses how often this activity-and-rest cycle of your heart takes place each minute. Physicians are concerned only when this basic life-sustaining rhythm is not in balance. A good strong heartbeat and pulse of blood through the body are signs of health to a physician, not a cause for worry.

Consider your breathing. The lungs fill with air as you inhale. When the lungs expand, they stretch the diaphragm, which is a sheetlike muscle above the abdomen. When the diaphragm is stretched, its natural tendency is to relax again. As it moves back to its relaxed position, air is gently pushed out of the lungs. They contract, and you exhale.

Expanding and contracting. Activity and rest. This is the principle polarity that maintains the equilibrium within all the systems of the natural world, whether we speak of the oceans, the seasons, our daily activities, or the organs of the body. This force that sustains life is self-generating. It need not be supervised. It is a force extending back to the beginning of time.

Distrusting the Unconscious

When I speak of the life-sustaining rhythm in the human body, I refer to it as being managed by the unconscious. My working definition of the word *unconscious* is "any part of the mind that we are not conscious of."

I needn't consciously remind myself to take my next breath or to have my next heartbeat. All the important functions of my body and mind are controlled unconsciously. I can certainly control the rhythm of my breathing consciously, but if I tried not to breathe, I wouldn't succeed. Even if I did a great job of holding my breath, I would eventually be forced to exhale or faint, allowing my unconscious to regain control.

When I sleep at night my conscious mind relinquishes complete control of my body to my unconscious. If I were injured and feeling severe pain I would probably faint (or "lose consciousness") while my unconscious regulated my essential bodily functions.

So, what am I leading up to? You are glad I like the ocean, you already know how long you work each day, and, yes, your heart beats regularly without constant reminders. What's the point?

The point is this: Panic erodes your basic trust in your body. Panic wins control over you by convincing you to doubt your body's natural *unconscious* monitoring system. Panic says, "Keep watching, keep listening, keep monitoring." These are the destructive messages of panic.

If you are constantly on guard over your body's sensations, you will need to start thinking about your body in a new way.

How do you allow yourself to fall asleep at night? Sure, you are exhausted from the day and you need your sleep. But when you fall asleep, you are no longer going to be able to consciously monitor your vital functions. You can't listen to your heartbeat, you can't make certain that you'll get the next breath of fresh air. What lets you relinquish that conscious control? What is it that you are implicitly trusting?

If you've found an answer, it's probably along the lines of "trusting that something would make sure my heart keeps pumping." Again, for simplicity's sake, let's label that something "the unconscious mind." What if, at the time of a panic attack, you could convince yourself to rely on that same unconscious to help you manage your body's sensations? I can guarantee that when you learn this skill you will be back in the driver's seat. You will no longer be letting panic have control, nor will you be forcing your conscious mind to do all the work. Instead, you will take full advantage of the remarkable control possible through a team effort. Your conscious thoughts will do half the work; your natural unconscious processes will do the rest.

As you may know, the unconscious has been viewed in the past as some dark and deep part of the psyche, full of painful traumas, and repressed emotions from childhood. In the past, psychoanalysis was seen as a decade-long process of dredging up these hidden memories by means of the patient's dreams and free associations. Its goal was to gain conscious insight and control over negative unconscious impulses.

This, I believe, is the wrong approach for coping with panic. The unconscious is ninety-nine percent brilliant in its ability to constantly direct the body toward health. For winning over panic attacks, the unconscious *needs no fixing* and *needs no supervision* by your conscious mind. It's perfectly fine. It simply needs to be permitted to do its work without intrusion. It is the conscious mind's intrusion that is the problem—that little voice that says, "What if these sensations get worse? Something bad will happen. Watch out!"

The Emergency Response

When I was living in Massachusetts, I once drove to the Outer Banks of North Carolina for a week's vacation at the ocean. This was the scenario as I was heading south.

· · ·

I am looking forward to being with my brother and his wife during that week on the beach, so part of my mind is drifting to images of playful times as I drive down Interstate 95. Another part of me is aware of how crowded the highway has become now that we are close to Philadelphia. I move to the outside lane to keep up speed. Driver's ed. classes teach us to keep a comfortable distance of one car length for each ten miles per hour. But today in this lane no one is thinking of such things. The task is to keep close to the car ahead of you so that no one else can squeeze in from the slower lane. You jockey for position and keep a heavy foot on the gas pedal. I'm cruising at just under sixty-five miles an hour, and no one's breaking in.

· · ·

Suddenly I see a small BMW three cars in front of me sharply swerve into the right lane and back again. In an instant the second car ahead of me swerves in a similar manner. My immediate thought is, "We're as good as dead. Here comes the crash." My eyes flash to the rearview mirror and back again. Just like a giant ripple in the stream of cars, the Chrysler ahead of me also veers out, almost hitting the truck to its right. And now I'm on top of it: a large eight-foot-long metal bumper, lying diagonally in front of my car, ready to slam into the left front tire. Before another thought registers in my mind, I veer out and back into my lane, circumventing death.

. . .

The thought of our demise seems to slow the pace of all of us in the fast lane. I let out a deep sigh and gradually merge into the right lane. My heart seems to be pumping out of my chest, my armpits are soaked, and I have a throbbing headache. I place my hand over my heart—partly to verify the pounding, partly to contain it.

Of course, I was not having a panic attack. My body and mind had just given a peak performance. Together, they had totally transformed their functions. The time between the instant that small BMW swerved and I veered past the bumper of the Chrysler in front of me was probably less than six seconds. In those moments, the pupils of my eyes dilated to improve their vision, absorbed in detail every movement of the cars in front of me, flashed to the rearview mirror to assess the distance and speed of the cars behind. Meanwhile, peripheral vision registered the vehicles to my right, and all this data was fed instantaneously to my brain. My hearing automatically became acutely sensitive to any relevant sounds. The blood flow to my hands and feet decreased and the excess blood was redirected to my deeper skeletal muscles. Blood also pooled in my torso to provide an abundance of nourishment to any vital organ in need during the emergency. My heart increased its pace to the degree necessary to get blood near my vital organs. My blood pressure thus increased. My breathing accelerated to provide for the increased oxygen needs of my rapidly circulating blood. That newly oxidized blood rushed to the brain, where the increased supply of oxygen stimulated my thought processes and significantly improved my reaction time. The muscles in my arms, hands, legs, and feet tensed in readiness for instructions from the brain and responded with precision. My liver released increased amounts of glucose (sugar) into the bloodstream to power my muscles and feed my brain and heart.

It is truly phenomenal, this body of ours. Nothing that humankind has ever created can come close to its performance. My conscious thought processes were not responsible for saving my life. Instead, they had one task: to prevent fear from interfering with the task. My life was in the hands of my autonomic nervous system, which signals the release of adrenaline and coordinates all efforts of the brain and the body with literally split-second timing.

Here are the major changes that take place in the body during such an Emergency Response:

- The blood sugar level increases.
- The pupils dilate.
- The sweat glands perspire.
- The heart rate increases.
- The muscles tense.
- The amount of blood in the hands and feet is reduced.
- The blood pools in the head and trunk.

These are normal, healthy, life-saving changes in the body's physiology, produced by communication from the brain to the autonomic nervous system, the endocrine system, and the motor nerves of the skeletal muscles. When the brain receives word that a crisis is at hand, it flips the "emergency" switch. All systems react simultaneously and instantly.

Tricking the Brain

In all likelihood, you have recognized some of these physiological changes as symptoms of panic. Your panic attacks are not identical to the body's natural, healthy Emergency Response. However, since this is a self-help book and not a medical textbook, I will take some liberties with the technical details. View it this way: anxiety attacks are produced when panic deceives the brain into believing there is imminent danger. There you are, standing in the aisle of the grocery store, not bothering a soul. Flip. On goes the emergency switch. "Red alert! All systems prepare for battle!" shouts the commanding voice of the brain, through the nervous system to the skeletal system, the muscles, the circulatory and respiratory systems, the endocrine system, and most organs of the body.

Since this is an unconscious response produced at an illogical time, you are consciously surprised and frightened. The reason you have more sensations than those I just listed is that panic now induces anxiety. Anxiety exaggerates the normal, healthy Emergency Response, and anxiety also feeds on itself. I said that during an Emergency Response the best thing for the conscious mind to do is to prevent fear or doubt from interfering with the task at hand. Panic, however, instructs you to focus on your body (*wrong!*) and worry about what will happen next (*wrong!*). Those two instructions are responsible for extreme sensations of anxiety that you experience during a panic attack. They can cause these changes:

- The heart may seem to skip a beat or beat irregularly.
- The stomach may feel as though it's tied in knots.
- The hands, arms, or legs may shake.
- You may have difficulty catching your breath.
- You may feel pains or tightness in your chest.
- The jaw, neck, or shoulders may feel tight and stiff.
- The mouth may become dry.
- You may have difficulty swallowing.
- The hands and feet may feel cold, sweaty, or numb.
- You may develop a headache.

Although several other changes are also possible (see Chapter 1), I list these here because they are all clearly exaggerations of the normal, healthy Emergency Response. For instance, during a crisis the autonomic nervous system—with its fight-flight-or-freeze response—produces what is called a "sympathetic stimulation" throughout the body, causing the sphincter muscles of the stomach to contract while blood flow to the digestive system is decreased. Anxiety will then increase the chance of heartburn, nausea, and pain in the upper abdomen and chest. In addition to exaggerating the normal physical changes of the body, making you focus your attention on your body and inviting you to worry about the future, panic produces a fourth problem: it prolongs your discomfort.

After a normal, healthy Emergency Response, the brain signals the end to the "sympathetic stimulation" of the nervous system. The body begins its swing back to "normal mode." Panic and anxiety, on the other hand, tend to let sensations linger. The headache throbs for the rest of the day, or the stomach churns through the night, disrupting your needed rest. The body feels depleted, exhausted; the mind seems to hang in a fog.

To summarize:

1. The human body and its organs, like those of all living organisms, maintain a balance between activity and rest, between expansion and contraction. A shifting from one of these poles to the other creates a healthy, natural rhythm.
2. The body is specially designed to handle extreme activity. It responds to an emergency automatically, through instinct. It is well equipped to perform at an instant's notice.
3. Panic disrupts the natural balance of the body by sending false emergency signals to the brain and by telling you to doubt your body's natural abilities.

To conquer panic attacks as they occur, you must know and believe the following:

1. You can trust your body and your unconscious to perform their essential roles during crises because the body has an Emergency Response.
2. When panic flips on the emergency switch, you can consciously flip it off.
3. With practice, you can consciously stop panic even before it takes control.

CHAPTER 9

Why the Body Reacts

If the brain is such a brilliant machine with an incredible capacity for intelligence, why doesn't it block out panic? Since it is the brain that signals all the physical sensations of panic, then the brain, as executive, must take responsibility for the failure.

To understand why the brain doesn't block out panic we must delve deeper into the workings of the mind and the brain. Most of the time I use the words *brain* and *mind* as synonyms, but occasionally they must be distinguished. I define the brain as the primary center for regulating and coordinating the body's activities. It also generates thought, memory, reason, emotion, and judgment. The brain is an actual physical object. The mind, on the other hand, is a concept, representing the ability to integrate the functions of the brain: perceiving our surroundings, experiencing our emotions, and processing information intelligently. In a sense, the brain is the work-horse of the mind. This is why I speak so much about altering your thoughts and beliefs. They are the keys to your brain's activity.

In a nutshell, here is what the brain does:

- It receives a stimulus.
- It interprets the meaning of that stimulus.
- It selects a response.
- It enlists the body to cooperate as needed.

For example, if you accidentally touch a hot radiator, (1) the stimulus travels up the nerve endings of your finger through the spinal cord to the brain, (2) the brain interprets the stimulus to mean "I'm touching something hot. This is burning and uncomfortable," (3) the brain selects to remove the finger from the radiator, and (4) it sends a communication through the nerves to the muscles in the arm, hand, and finger. Your hand instantly jerks away.

You might consider it an instinctual response to jerk your hand off a hot object. It is also a learned response. The early experiences of your life, dating back to infancy, have trained your brain to interpret contact with a hot radiator in that manner.

The brain interprets sensations on the basis of two criteria: memory- and sensory-based images. Significant events of your life are recorded in memory-based images with varying degrees of intensity. I have a distinct memory of poking a stick in a small fire when I was four years old. That memory is reinforced through a sensory-based image: the smell of the burning lumber, the sight of those flames, the touch of my hand on that stick. Interestingly, I don't have an image of that stick breaking, causing me to fall into coals. My next memory is of sitting on the counter of my neighbor's kitchen. I can see several adults around me, feel the ointment covering the minor burns on my knees, and recall the grown-ups offering me a soft drink.

These events live on in memory, reinforced by sensory-based images. The actual event is not the only thing recorded in the memory. In addition, our internal reactions are etched in our unconscious mind. A few minutes before I fell into that fire, my mother had instructed my six-year-old brother and me to "stay away from that fire." So in addition to the immediate pain I experienced from the burns, I suspect that in my memory I also hold the sense of guilt I must have felt for disobeying.

Well-worn Paths

Our beliefs and values develop largely out of our life experiences and the memories of them. As adults, all of us probably notice that certain patterns and habits stem from our childhood experiences. Such things as our religious beliefs, our social skills, our use or abuse of alcohol, our choice of partners, are based in part on our childhood memories and in part on past adult experiences.

This past learning is of tremendous benefit to us today. So many decisions are simple for us because we already have the "circuits" in place. We don't need to put much conscious effort into remembering our phone number or writing a letter or tying a ribbon on a package. But as children, learning each of these skills was a challenge. Can you remember? As we mastered each skill, we literally created new neurological circuits in our brain, circuits that we have now used for years. They become like well-worn paths. Every time we learn new skills, we create new circuits.

But with every positive there seems to be a negative. Here is the rub: strong beliefs can *block* the natural protective mechanisms of the brain and mind. Left to its own, the unconscious mind will seek health. But social learning and certain traumatic experiences tend to override the unconscious mind.

After the panic response is established, the mind stops working creatively in your favor. Instead it seems to be set on "automatic pilot" and stops seeking out solutions. The mind focuses on the problem instead of on its solution. When you walk into a situation that is similar in time or place to one in which you previously had a panic attack, the image of that last time rises up in your mind. This image alone can produce the same muscle tension and the mind can interpret it to mean "trouble." Instead of paying attention to all of its many problem-solving options, the mind focuses on its negative images of your past failure. In turn, you begin to notice your tense muscles and all of your other disturbing body sensations.

A panic attack may completely surprise you—consciously. But unconsciously a step-by-step process has taken place prior to your physical sensations:

Step 1: When you enter a situation that is associated with panic, the brain registers this stimulus.

Step 2: It interprets the meaning of this stimulus as "harmful" or "dangerous."

Step 3: On the basis of your memory of past experiences, your brain doubts your ability to cope effectively.

Step 4: It therefore selects "emergency" as its default response, compounded by "anxiety" (since it doubts that you will cope well).

Step 5: The brain enlists the body in the Emergency Response. After enough of those experiences, you develop a conditioned response, meaning the brain takes less and less time to evaluate each new situation. Instead, it automatically selects the Emergency Response. You have created a "well-worn path." The mind then takes that specific threat and generalizes it. This explains why people who have their first panic attack in a car may gradually develop a fear of any form of transportation. The brain stops screening the stimulus. If a person has a panic attack in a restaurant, bank, or other closed space, eventually the mind might say, "All such situations are dangerous."

Images and Interpretations

Images can produce brain responses just as well as the actual experiences do, and this creates further limitations. If you have experienced panic during public speaking in the past, simply the *image* of seeing yourself giving a talk next week can produce uncomfortable feelings right now. In your fantasy of the future you imagine having a rough time of it. You don't call up a view of yourself standing in front of the group, organized and prepared, feeling confident, speaking distinctly, being well received by your audience. Instead, you envision yourself in front of the group, then you ask yourself, "What if I begin to panic?" That suggestion triggers an image of you panicking during your speech. And right now, one week before the event, you begin to have those physical sensations that you expect to have during the event. This is an example of the powerful tools of the mind.

Here is a key point. Much of your ability to control anxiety attacks is based on this principle: People, places, events are panic-provoking only *after* we apply meaning to them. A store is just a store, a speech is just a speech, a drive is just a drive, until the brain interprets them as "dangerous" or "threatening." To conquer panic, then, you must intervene at the *point of interpretation*.

Taking Away Choice

There are two reasons why the brain selects the Emergency Response at inappropriate times. The first is that it is prevented from gathering relevant information in the present moment. Many of our observations and beliefs about life were established during our youth, well before our adult intellect was mature. Other beliefs were formed after fearful moments or traumatic events. When these beliefs are fixed in place, they prevent the brain from evaluating new situations with an "open mind," so to speak. Once a belief about threat is established, the mind won't constantly reevaluate the facts associated with the belief. When beliefs are useful ("Hot objects can burn you"), we benefit. But when a faulty belief is in place ("All forms of transportation are dangerous to me"), our lives become restricted and uncreative.

If you suffer from panic attacks, it means that a faulty belief prevents your brain from receiving a critical message. Remember steps 1 and 2 of all brain activity during threat. At Step 1 the brain receives a stimulus (e.g., entering a restaurant or thinking of giving a speech) and at Step 2 it interprets the stimulus. It is at Step 2 that the brain is missing a message. The faulty belief of "This is an emergency!" prevents an accurate interpretation of the situation, namely, "There is *no physical danger*." The brain doesn't bother to look around this new scene, gathering information to make an assessment. Instead, it receives an immediate message that forces the Emergency Response.

Another reason the brain selects the Emergency Response is by default: it doesn't know of another, more appropriate response. From an evolutionary standpoint, the human intellect is a relatively recent development, when compared to the Emergency Response, which is also found in all lower animals. Perhaps our intellectual and psychological defenses have not evolved adequately enough to handle certain social threats, so our physical defenses respond instead. The fact remains that the Emergency Response produces a handful of significant changes in the body strictly designed to help in a physical crisis, yet actually handicap us in dealing with social or intellectual challenges. Most of us can imagine the difficulty in trying to pass a final exam in mathematics while the hands sweat, the mouth dries, and the muscles tense.

You have intellectual and psychological capabilities that can reverse this intrusion of the Emergency Response. This book tells you how to identify these capacities, how to master them, and how to use them to take control of panic. Your first task is to work on changing your interpretation of events. Over a period of time you must slowly reinforce this message: You are not confronting an emergency. Sooner or later it will be one of the messages you tell yourself at the moment you sense panic creeping in. Eventually it will become one of the automatic, unconscious interpretations of your brain: "This is not an emergency."

It is perfectly fine for you to become highly alert and experience an increase in your heart rate and respiration during a panic-provoking situation. These responses are positive and mean that you will have the capacity to think more sharply and clearly. As you face these fearful times and places, clear, sharp thinking will be your ally. Your goal should not be to eliminate all these sensations. A certain amount of anxiety and worry can be beneficial. In research comparing the test scores of students who enter exams completely relaxed, somewhat anxious, or very anxious, the students who were somewhat anxious performed the best. When we anticipate an event with excitement or anxiety, the adrenal glands secrete hormones that stimulate our creative intelligence, which we will need when facing such events. This same process takes place when you face panic. The goal is to keep your alertness while you change your interpretation. That alertness gives you a conscious choice, so that you don't have to respond with your old automatic fears.

You will now learn a series of strategies that allows you to remain alert and sharp to all that is taking place around you and within you, while at the same time consciously flipping off that emergency switch. With practice, you will be able to consciously stop panic before it begins.

The healthy mental processes of our brains are so closely tied to the functioning of our bodies during threat that I am going to introduce a short-hand term for their relationship. Throughout the rest of the book you will see the term *body-&-mind,* and I will identify it in the singular instead of the plural. This will refer to our unconscious thought patterns and the signals that the brain passes on to the body. Each person's body-&-mind is well-trained through genetics and life experience. If panic has intruded into your life, we can assume it has been manipulating your body-&-mind.

But that can change and *will* change if you can follow these guidelines. All my recommended strategies will be grounded in a great respect for the ability of the body-&-mind to return to its natural, healthy state of adaptability.

Don't Panic *Live*:

PART III

Your Moment-by-Moment Strategies

CHAPTER 10

Grab a New Attitude

How does one fight anxiety attacks?

I am sitting in Linda M.'s living room, listening to the story of her six-year battle with panic. The curtains are drawn, as if to keep out the fear. After the first year of struggle she remained behind the doors of her home, too afraid to step outside.

> As soon as I consider taking a walk alone, my heart begins to pound and I get a tingling feeling from my upper body right down to my knees and toes. It feels as if my throat will close. I can't swallow. I try to fight all these symptoms at once, but that seems to bring on the panic. The more I fight it, the worse I become. I ask myself the same questions: "What's making me this way? Why does it continue? Why does it get worse?"

Donna B., whom we met in Chapter 4, is an agoraphobic who has suffered from anxiety attacks for twenty-one years. During her worst months only her bedroom was a safe haven from her fears.

When that panicky feeling starts, I want to fight it. But instead I almost always run from it. And it seems the faster I run, the faster it catches up to me. I've used the expression "quicksand": the more I struggle, the deeper I sink into it. After a while I almost feel the surrender: 'OK, fear, you've got me.'"

Linda and Donna fight the most devastating form of panic—the extreme case in which the individual becomes trapped inside her own home. Yet they illustrate the two primary ways each of us tends to battle our enemies. If we must face them, we gather our resources to fight them head-to-head. If we feel inadequately prepared to fight and win, we choose to steer clear of them to avoid any kind of confrontation. With panic these two strategies seem to fail. As Linda describes, the more you fight the uncomfortable sensations directly, the stronger they seem to grow.

The more you run from panic, the faster it seems to chase you. The more you avoid panic-provoking situations, the more panic controls your life. If we place ourselves on guard, waiting and watching for the next signs of trouble, we are inviting panic to return sooner. How? By establishing a special relationship with panic, a relationship of opposites.

Our instinctual defenses fail to overcome panic. In fact, they actually support the recurrence of anxiety attacks. We encourage and strengthen the power of panic by treating it as our "enemy," to be avoided or to be battled. To take control of panic you need to understand this special relationship and then learn how to alter it. Let's look closely at this paradoxical change in stance toward anxiety and how to apply it during the moment of panic.

The Balance of Power

All the activities of our world are built around a dynamic tension between opposing forces. In Chapter 8 I described the balance between rest and activity and between expansion and contraction; using the examples of the ocean tides, a pendulum, summer and winter, day and night, our patterns of work and rest, and the movements of our heart and lungs. I presented them as essential life-sustaining rhythms. The Emergency Response—the alarm system in our body-&-mind—has an equally powerful and opposing system that quiets and calms us. (I will detail this Calming Response in Chapter 16.) It seems logical that the body-&-mind has a way of bringing crisis back into balance.

Polarity creates and maintains all types of activity. Every book, play, short story, movie, or TV show involves at least one basic polarity: antagonist versus protagonist, a detective missing the answers, a man wanting a woman, a teenager struggling between right and wrong, a poor family seeking food or shelter. Without this basic push-and-pull found in conflict, desire, struggle, decisions, or other differences, these dramas would not succeed. It is the tension of unresolved problems that maintains our interest and involvement. In world politics, major activity is found only where polarity exists, such as ideological differences between the United States and the Soviet Union from the 1960s through the 1980s or one country's need to import what it is missing and another's need to export what the other needs.

On a more personal level, all parents have experienced this same dynamic when they take a toy away from a child; instantly the struggle begins because now the child *wants* the toy. If you surrender and give the toy back, the child is soon bored with it and moves to some other activity. Scientifically, opposites attract. Place the north end of a bar magnet next to another magnet. It will repel the other north end and attach itself to the south end. To make sure we continue to populate the earth, Mother Nature creates men and women as attractive opposites, producing desire.

In each of these examples there exists a complementary relationship between two opposites. Think of your own life and the lives of others around you. Whenever we set our minds to a goal, whether it is to graduate from school, achieve recognition, cook a meal, or take a vacation, we create this dynamic tension by choosing something we don't already have. We produce our positive, goal-oriented drive by distinguishing between what we have now and what we want. We are missing that degree, that recognition, that supper, or that vacation. And we seek out what we are missing. Once we reach that goal, we stop working and come to rest. Of course, moments later we have some new goal, large or small, because this process takes place constantly. These polarities, and the ensuing tensions they create, are not bad or wrong; in fact, they are the driving force of all action. If activity is taking place within a given field, you will find a basic tension between two opposites.

Now let's reverse the tables. How do you write a screenplay that will fail at the box office? Here is one way: make all your characters happy and content. Don't let any character worry or set a tough goal for himself or realize that he needs something more in his life. Let no one struggle to fulfill a dream. How will your audience react? *Zzzzz*.

How might we reduce the hostile tensions between two opposing countries? We could discover a foe that is more powerful than either country alone (a worldwide disaster, another Hitler, or aliens from outer space). This would shift the dynamic tension toward a new polarity, a new "them versus us."

How could you make yourself depressed? By never setting any goals for yourself, by never striving toward the future. By not believing that things change or that you can change. By expecting that tomorrow will turn out just as badly as yesterday did. How could you deepen your depression? By creating a polarity in your mind between "everybody else" (who can change) and you (who can never be different).

How to Invite Panic

In light of this principle of tension between opposites, how might panic attacks continue in someone's life? *Whenever you resist something, that something will persist,* because you have created a polarity. By resisting a panic attack, you support it, and the stronger your resistance, the greater your support.

Think of how you currently respond to your fear of having an anxiety attack. You struggle. You avoid. You try to control the outcome of events. The essence of your reaction is, "I don't want that." Such a statement reflects your current attitude toward anxiety: "It's bad. It's wrong. I'm inadequate for having it. It has to go away for me to be OK." You also resist the possible effects of that anxiety: "I can't let people see me this way. I don't want to lose my concentration again. It would be awful if I have to walk out of this meeting."

Here are several ways to prolong the existence of panic in your life:

- Fear panic
- Actively fight against a panic attack
- Avoid any panic-provoking situation
- Set a goal of "never ever" having another anxiety attack
- Worry about the next time you might feel the sensations of panic
- Try not to notice tensions
- Expect to master panic before you face it again
- Run away from panic sensations

Each of these actions invites anxiety attacks by creating a dynamic tension between you and panic. This tension provides the energy that sustains the process. You must interrupt this pattern if you are going to take control. Here is the paradox: To win against panic you must stop fighting it or running away from it.

- What do you say when you start getting anxious? "I don't want that!"
- And if you think the anxiety will continue? "I can't handle that!"
- What about the possibility of your anxiety getting stronger? "I don't want that!"
- How about the thought of having an actual panic attack? "I *certainly* don't want that!"

Since you typically know the circumstances that cause you to get anxious and panicky, then you also resist and avoid them:

- *Feeling physically trapped.* Can you imagine standing in front of the open door of a crowded elevator, about to step in, and anticipating that anxious, closed-in feeling? What do you say to yourself? "I don't want that!"
- *Feeling socially trapped.* When your friend asks you to lunch, and you fear you might be nervous around her, how do you react? "I don't want that!"
- *Not knowing what will happen next.* How about the possibility of spending the night in a hotel alone, out of town, when you aren't sure how anxious you might become in that setting? "I can't handle that!"
- *Acting "incompetently" in public.* As you anticipate any social situation, do you imagine getting visibly lost and confused or people hearing your voice shake? "I don't want that! I can't cope with it!"

Notice when you resist or avoid a specific set of circumstances, you do so because you think the circumstances will increase the likelihood of any of these outcomes:

- You'll get anxious
- Your anxiety will continue

- Your anxiety will get stronger
- You might have a panic attack or some other negative consequence

You are not willing to have any of these experiences. That seems logical; who in their right mind would want any of that! Yet there is a problem, because to recover from panic, *you must embrace all those possible outcomes.* Crazy, but true. That's why we call this process paradoxical: it is opposite of logic. Are you familiar with this adage? "Anything that is resisted will persist." Your resistance—your commitment to fight or avoid your discomfort—actually *causes* your continual problems with panic.

Here is what I know to be true after almost 30 years of treating people with panic disorder: resisting and avoiding will *keep* panic in your life. If you are currently suffering from panic attacks, it is likely that you can simply enter a situation and become panicky without much of a thought. To stay anxious in that situation probably means you are sensing a continued threat. *That is to be expected.* Your body-&-mind will react to threat with the Emergency Response—the fight-flight-or-freeze response of autonomic arousal. If you aren't certain how you will manage that situation, then worried thoughts will rise up spontaneously. *That is also normal.* What we need to pay attention to is your reaction to that reaction. Do you now continue to make statements that support your threatened feelings? "If this goes like last time, I'm going to be miserable here. I can't tolerate that again. I have to stop it from happening. Maybe I should take another anti-anxiety pill. Maybe I should just get out of here." These are the kinds of messages we want to change. In a threatening situation, you are *not* in control of what pops up automatically from your body-&-mind: your initial physical anxiety and your initial fearful thoughts. What you *are* in control of is your next response.

Get Inoculated Against Panic

How do you recover from such a powerful and painful pattern? How do you stop fighting panic or running away from it?

Every year that I work with people having panic attacks I become more convinced that you have one *primary* task: to manage your attitude. You control anxiety attacks by changing your attitude about them. Attitude means your basic view of your relationship with panic and anxiety, your judgment of panic, your belief about how you should act in the face of anxiety. Consider it synonymous with disposition, point of view, relationship, stance, mindset. Once you start thinking about anxiety, your attitude will direct of all your actions.

Since I want you to absorb this message, let me say it again: The single most important way to win over panic attacks is to respond to them from a different point of view. To get better, you don't struggle with anxiety, you don't try to get rid of the uncomfortable sensations, you don't avoid threatening situations. You choose to take a different attitude toward them. With this new attitude in place, you will know what actions to take.

As we approach any task, our attitudes and beliefs influence the degree to which we are willing to try to solve problems, our determination to persist in the face of obstacles and the amount of time and energy we devote to the endeavor. So, pay attention to all the skills in this book, and practice the skills regularly. Review the facts on any special areas of interest to you. Follow the step-by-step guidelines that I offer. But when you are ready to take on panic, focus primarily on your attitude. That will be the driving force of your healing.

Few self-help books put most of their emphasis on attitude. Typically they will direct you to make lists of your strengths, prioritize your goals, experiment with new behaviors, and record your changes. These are excellent suggestions for a self-help approach, but it is the nature of *panic* that requires you to go beyond technique to modifying your attitude. I firmly believe—

after talking with thousands of people in treatment sessions, training programs, and public lectures—that it is attitude, not technique, that will take you across the finish line.

Consider the possibility that you can "inoculate" yourself with a new set of attitudes. One of the greatest achievements in medicine began when William Jenner discovered that fluid from cowpox sores could immunize people against the deadly disease of smallpox. Physicians can now inoculate against dozens of illnesses, from polio, rubella, and yellow fever to tetanus, hepatitis B, and rabies.

A vaccine consists of a dead or modified form of a disease-causing microbe. Once injected, it stimulates the body's production of antibodies to the microbe. If the microbe should subsequently enter the body, the antibodies help neutralize and remove the microbe from the body before it can multiply and cause disease. You inoculate yourself by taking in some of the causative agent in order to experiment with it or to become immune to it. Therefore, inoculations are paradoxical treatments: *They take you close to the threat.*

What attitude should you have?

One that contradicts what your instinct tells you

One that is exactly opposite of the reaction that every fiber in your body and every cell in your brain urges you to have

One that is counter to how you truly believe you should respond

One that you won't like much!

How do you inoculate yourself against anxiety attacks? Go directly toward panic, drop your guard, and freely choose to let it touch you. Wow! That is a crazy idea! I'm going to do my best to persuade you that this is *exactly* what you need to do to recover, then I will outline how to practice applying this stance as a skill. When you master it, you will incorporate a set of attitudes that will guide your future. They will sound like this: "I'll become stronger by purposely facing what I am afraid of. I want to do that, and I can handle it." Then you will be immune to panic, which means not being affected by it or reactive to it.

How valuable can your attitude be? I know many people who have applied *no* techniques—they didn't control their breathing, they didn't learn relaxation skills, they didn't plan strategies for coping with uncomfortable sensations—and they still brought their panic under control in a matter of weeks. They did that by focusing strictly on the attitudes presented in this section of the book.

The reverse is not true. I have known many more people who have attempted to apply techniques without a shift in their attitude. They tried on the skills while simultaneously thinking, "This better work! I can't stand this anxiety. I shouldn't be feeling this way." Unfortunately, they continued to struggle with the discomforts of anxiety and panic.

Love the Mat

The martial arts, developed in Asia, teach self-discipline, physical combat technique, and a philosophy, or attitude, about life. All but one are ancient schools. Aikido, a twentieth-century martial art based on love and dedicated to peace, puts a different spin on the art of self-defense. And "spin" is an appropriate expression. In the Western world, we use boxing as the prototype for fighting. If someone punches, you punch back. You meet force with opposing force. By contrast, the traditional martial arts axiom is "Push when pulled and pull when pushed." As the attacker approaches you to push or punch, you learn to grab the forward moving hand and pull it. You don't oppose the challenger with equal force. You take the attacker's movement and energy and use it against him. For instance, as he pushes, you pull him past you and onto the ground.

In Aikido the axiom "Push when pulled and pull when pushed" becomes "turn when pushed and enter when pulled." You accept, join, and move with the challenger's energy flow in the direction it is going. You offer nothing for the challenger to resist. You turn and spin with the attacker instead of moving past him.

Learning the art of Aikido requires *sincerely welcoming* the attack and struggle, *truly understanding* the attacker's intentions, and *loving* the attacker. The moment the challenger begins to approach with an attack, the Aikido student shifts her position. She stands with open arms and open palms, "welcoming" the challenger. If you try it for a moment, holding your arms out by your side with your palms open to the front, you will notice how vulnerable you feel.

I will leave the details of other Aikido moves to the masters. It is the basic attitude that I want to address. The attitudinal stance in Aikido is that *each challenge holds within it an opportunity* to learn and practice. The student views the challenge as a gift of energy, a creative system of joining rather than one of conflict. This view eliminates the notion of "enemy." They are not ignoring the facts of the situation—"a fist is moving rapidly toward my face and may soon make impact." But they train themselves to rapidly grab an attitude that directs their response, so that they will automatically override any poor defensive strategies.

Another common expression in the martial arts is "Love the mat." During the learning process you'll find yourself again and again lying flat out on the mat after your opponent gets the best of you. By embracing challenging experiences as a necessary part of your training, you reduce your resistance to the learning process. "Love the mat" is a winning attitude of students who know that they don't always get to be in control.

Many people make the error of designing practice sessions in which they enter the fearful situations *until the point* that they feel discomfort. Then they retreat. This approach makes their recovery process long and arduous.

The only way to get the best of panic is to face discomfort directly and willingly. The task of provoking your discomfort—loving the mat—requires courage. Think of courage as "being scared and doing it anyway." This way, as you face panic, you don't have to *get rid* of fear, you need to *add* courage. In fact, you only need courage in fearful situations!

Provoking your discomfort is exactly what I am going to encourage you to do in the coming pages. I'll be asking you to set up events that will provoke your distress. Some would say that this goes beyond courage to stupidity. It's like being in the jungle and running *toward* the lion's roar. But that is the move, and the expression "run toward the roar" will be a useful reminder.

The nature of panic is that it produces involuntary sensations in your body. By voluntarily seeking out those sensations you begin to change panic. You take away its involuntary nature and start to shift the control over to you. So as you accept this challenge of "I want to face my discomfort," remember to "love the mat" and "run toward the roar."

The approach we are going to take in these next chapters will help you learn, over time, to perceive situations as less threatening. By now in the book you should know that the physical sensations you experience are uncomfortable but are normal and not harmful. Yet until your body-&-mind is trained to know that too, it will generate fear when you get uncomfortable. Likewise, if you predict that you will make mistakes in an upcoming event, your body-&-mind will respond to your message—"I might perform poorly here, so this is a threatening situation"—by making you more apprehensive. *You cannot prevent those reactions yet,* because your body-&-mind will always go on guard when you communicate "danger" to it.

So what do you change? You start this project by changing how you react to what you notice. When you approach situations that scare you, then take on two new attitudes. First, it's normal to feel anxious in threatening situations. And, second, go *toward* the perceived threat. Now let's add three additional points of view to support this paradoxical stance toward anxiety. They are: "I'm going to drop my guard against anxiety," "I can handle this," and "I want this."

Drop Your Guard

Panic leads people to become vigilant. A panic attack hits suddenly, catches you by surprise, and generates your sense of threat. Our body-&-mind has been trained over hundreds of thousands of years to guard against harm. Toddlers don't have to burn themselves on a stove too many times before their built-in instinct trains them to watch out for stovetops. In that same way, when you've been "burned" several times by panic, your mind searches rapidly for danger signals anytime you approach a panic-provoking situation. You are watching, feeling, listening with great attention, on guard in case something "goes wrong" in your body or your surroundings. Unfortunately, all this vigilance only contributes to your distress. You are tensing yourself up in anticipation of a problem. This is the definition of anticipatory anxiety.

What about when a panic attack begins? Think about what you say to yourself. Even during panic, almost all your communications are anticipatory in nature: "I'm really feeling bad right now. *What if this gets worse?* I'm light-headed and dizzy. What if I faint *in a moment*? My face feels flushed. *What if people start seeing this?*" On and on it goes. "I can't let myself *get any worse.* I can't let the symptoms *increase.*" You project yourself ahead, into a potentially worsening situation, and the effects are logical: you become more anxious and worried.

This natural, instinctual response to threat works against you. When you stay on guard as you approach events, you increase your tension and become more vulnerable to a panic attack. When you warn yourself to stay on guard in the midst of panic, you secrete even greater amounts of adrenaline into your bloodstream, causing more intense sensations. You can't remain anxiously on guard and simultaneously learn to control panic.

Most problems with anxiety relate to a fear of uncertainty. My educated guess is that the brain chemistry of about 20 percent of the population leads them to have a more difficult time than the average person in tolerating *uncertainty regarding risk*. Of course, this can put them at a disadvantage, since living demands risk. It is no wonder, then, that so many people develop anxiety problems. They worry because their brain is demanding closure on a specific issue. Their mind says, "This is how it must turn out for me to feel secure. And I must feel secure. Do I know for certain it will turn out this way?" It is as though they require a one-hundred percent guarantee that they will encounter zero risk. That is simply too much to ask of life. If you intend to go up against one of the most powerful forces of the natural world—continual change—you will have a tough time winning. Listen to these expectations of life and you will see what I mean. The person with panic attacks, phobias, or social anxieties asks questions such as:

"Can I know for certain that I won't have any symptoms?"
"Can I know for certain that I won't have to leave?"
"Can I know for certain that I won't feel trapped?"
"Can I know for certain that this isn't a heart attack?"
"Can I know for certain that I won't die on that plane?"
"Can I know for certain that I won't cause an embarrassing scene?"
"Can I know for certain that people won't stare at me?"
"Can I know for certain that I won't have a panic attack?"

If we look at a different anxiety problem—obsessive-compulsive disorder—we find the same kinds of questions:

"Am I sure that this object is clean?"

"Am I sure that I won't get contaminated if I touch the ground?"

"Am I sure that my family will be safe?"

"Am I sure that I didn't run someone over?"

"Am I sure that I unplugged that iron?"

"Am I sure that I won't kill my child?"

If you feel a strong yet inappropriate need for certainty, then confronting that problem will require that you challenge those demanding I-must-know thoughts. You will need to confront them consistently and directly *every day* to produce the change we want. This is where your new attitude comes in. You must find ways to accept risk and tolerate uncertainty.

Stay with me as I explain how this works, because this stance doesn't seem very attractive at first glance. Whatever outcome you fear, work to find a way to *accept that outcome as a possibility*. For example, imagine that sometimes when you begin to have panicky symptoms you feel a pain in your chest that runs down your left arm. Each time it happens, your first thought is, "This could be a heart attack!" Of course you have had one or more medical evaluations by a specialist. Let's also say that all physicians you consult declare that you have a strong heart, take proper care of yourself, and are not at risk of a heart attack.

Nonetheless, as soon as that pain shoots down your arm, you say, "This time it really could be my heart! How do I know? There's no guarantee that this is only panic. And if it is a heart attack, I need help now!"

Let's also say that you've been learning to reassure yourself as a way to get some perspective on panic. "OK . . . I've been to the emergency room twelve times in the last two years. One hundred percent of those visits have been false alarms. I know that I suffer from panic attacks, and this is what they feel like, too. Let me take a few calming breaths, relax and wait a few minutes. I'll begin to feel better."

The reassurance lasts all of five seconds. Then you start again. "But I don't *know*. I don't know *for certain*. If this is a heart attack I could die! Right *now*! There's always a chance."

It's the same with people's fear of dying on a plane. Commercial flight is the safest mode of transportation we have. On average, about 100 people in the United States die on a plane per year, while 47,000 motorists die on the highways and 8,000 pedestrians are killed each year. If you are looking for a risk-free environment, don't stay at home; 22,000 people in the United States die of accidents each year without even leaving their houses.

Even though your odds of dying on a plane are one in 7.5 million, the dialogue goes like this, "There's still a chance I might die. And if I do, that will be the most horrible, terrifying death I can imagine." You reassure yourself, "Planes are safe. You'll be fine. The pilot has gray hair; he has twenty-five years' experience." You counter, "Yes, but how do I *know*? How can I be *certain*?"

This is what you do to yourself, in your own unique areas of worry. You ask, "How can I be certain someone won't criticize me?" or "How can I be certain I won't have to leave the concert?" You might as well give it up, because you can never satisfy the demand for absolute confidence. No amount of reassurance will ever be enough. That demand is how you trap yourself. Here, instead, is the attitude to strive for: "I accept the possibility of a heart attack [plane crash/panic attack] happening."

> For fear of heart attacks: "I accept the possibility that this time it could actually be a heart attack. I'm going to respond to it as though it is a panic attack. I accept the risk that I might be wrong."
>
> For fear of dying on a plane: "I accept the possibility that this plane could crash. I'm going to think and feel and act as though this plane is one hundred percent safe. I accept the risk that I might be wrong."

For fear of having to leave an event: "I accept the pos-
bility that I might have to leave the restaurant. I imagine I'd feel embarrassed, but I'm willing to tolerate
that now."

By making the decision to accept the possibility of a negative
outcome, you circumvent the requirement for absolute certainty
of your future comfort and safety. There's always a chance you
will have a heart attack, regardless of your health. There's always a chance you could die in a plane crash, regardless of the
relative safety of air travel. There's always a chance you will
leave the restaurant and become embarrassed.

If you want to lower your chances of panicking and raise your
chances of flying comfortably or feeling more at ease at the restaurant, you have work to do. Your job is to lower your risk of
problems as much as makes common sense, then accept the remaining risk that is not under your control. You only have two
other basic options. You can keep worrying about the risk while
you continue with these behaviors. That option gives you more
anxiety and increases the likelihood of panic. Or you can withdraw from these activities. The world can get by with you never
flying again. The world can get by if you never enter another restaurant. There are consequences to this option, of course. (It
may take longer to travel to your friends or relatives, and so
forth.) But it's your choice.

I assume that these two options—worrying and avoiding—
have been your close friends for a while now, and yet here you
sit, reading this book, looking for alternative choices. There is a
better way to take control of anxiety attacks. I encourage you to
practice this idea of dropping your guard and accepting uncertainty and discover the rewards.

As I've mentioned, there is an interesting outcome of the
best therapeutic interventions designed to help you control anxiety: they actually make you more anxious at first. This one—
giving up the requirement for complete confidence in the

outcome—is a good example. For instance, imagine you begin to feel that pain in your chest that shoots down your left arm. Now you are saying, "I'm going to apply all my skills as though this is a panic attack. I'm not going to act as though this is a heart attack." Do you think one hundred percent of you is going to agree to this plan? No way! Some part of your mind is still going to feel scared, because, try as you might, that part of you will still be worried about a heart attack. Worrying, or fearful monitoring, is one of our most common ways to stay in control. If you practice letting go of your worries, your body-&-mind will feel somewhat out of control. That will make you anxious. This anxiety is the distress of positive experimentation and change; it's a good kind of anxiety. But expect it to be uncomfortable at first! Have faith that, over time, this anxiety will diminish.

The well-respected psychologist, Dr. Daniel Goleman once wrote, "A person prevails over anxiety by sacrificing attention." To come out on top you must let down your guard. You must not pay such close attention to what might happen next. You must clear your head of its constant and frantic analysis.

If you stop being so vigilant, you also run the risk that something might slip past your conscious attention. Some little twinge in your body could go unnoticed. Or, you might get stuck in a traffic jam before you think to exit the highway. This is another reason dropping your guard can make you feel more anxious at first, not less. When in the past you have kept your guard up as a way to stay in control, I am suggesting that you now let down your guard. If you do this, you may feel that you are not protecting yourself. When you feel vulnerable, you'll feel anxious. This is a good reason to become a student of the attitude, "It's OK to be anxious here."

When you decide to enter a threatening situation, it is fine to plan out how you will take care of yourself. But make those plans with the expectation that you may become anxious and not with the fearful dread that panic might strike. Include in those plans your decision to accept any anxiety as it arises, without holding yourself in a death grip waiting for its arrival. Your body-&-mind will best learn its new skills if you will allow anxiety to surprise you. The paradox to play with is *plan and don't stay on guard*.

If you will courageously practice these skills—turning your attention away from fearful analysis of every new stimulus and away from predictions of things going terribly wrong, being willing to be surprised by a problem arising, tolerating the anxiety of "not knowing," then you can turn your attention back to your valued tasks. Over time, you will learn the value of the attitude "I don't need to stay on guard against panic."

"I Can Handle This"

Imagine this scene. As you are walking into a room, you notice that you suddenly become physically anxious. You spontaneously think, "Oh, no, here comes anxiety. This is not a good time to get anxious." Now you notice you are even more anxious, because you just gave yourself a threatening message ("Oh, no, this is not good.")

OK . . . so . . . as absurd as this sounds, imagine at that moment you say to yourself and *believe,* the following message: "This is exactly what I want. I've been looking for another chance to be anxious. Now it's here. Good. I can handle this."

What is the effect of such a message, delivered honestly? I can probably guarantee that your anxiety won't disappear. However, you will be introducing a new attitude that will compete with your resisting stance of, "I don't want this! I can't handle it!"

What is required to handle a situation? There are two skills that most people with panic attacks need to master. The first is to assess the likelihood of a negative event. Here's how you might respond to your momentary worries about your health: "Really? I'm going to have a stroke now because I am so anxious? That's not what Dr. Chalmers says. I'm not falling for this one again. I'm anxious, but not in danger. I'm going to stick it out." The second is a willingness to tolerate the possibility of those events. If they are relatively unlikely events, you might say something like, "According to probability theory, I'd have to fly every single day for 26,000 years before I would die on a plane flight. I'm willing to take that chance to get over my panic disorder; I'm going on that flight." With the more likely outcomes, you might say, "Would I bother people if I had to get up in the middle of the symphony and walk out? Probably a few would be annoyed. But I can handle that if it happens. So I'm going to the symphony."

Here is the ideal position to aim for in any threatening situation: "No matter what happens, I'll figure out how to cope with it." Why have this attitude? Because you want a belief that supports you going *forward*, into the scene, not one that instructs you to back away. I don't have the room in these pages to review every possible scenario and suggest ways you can cope with it; this is going to be your independent responsibility. If you want to get better, then this is one of the best ways to help yourself: when events don't match your ideal outcome, commit to finding ways to tolerate that.

Could you go to a party and become so anxious that you have to excuse yourself in the middle of a conversation and head into the bathroom to cool out and re-group? Sure. That's certainly possible for any of us. The question is, could you handle it? Could you endure being embarrassed? Could you tolerate someone leaving the party thinking, "I wonder what was going on with her?" If your answer is "no," then you will continue to avoid. To get stronger, you will need to find ways to cope with such a possible outcome. Your power will come from your willingness to bounce back after an incident like that.

Could you get so anxious at the barbershop that you feel like you can't catch your breath, that you have to get up, with the bib still around your neck, while the barber is still cutting your hair, and walk out and drive home without paying? That is probably an unlikely event, but it certainly would be embarrassing. And you could do it. You would survive, and you would piece yourself back together. But you will need to strengthen your belief that you could manage that unpleasant event, or you won't go forward.

When you get anxious about being trapped, panic will generate such unlikely scenarios and scare you with such outcomes. If they are realistic possibilities, the question is, could you cope with them? Could you tolerate the barber being caught off guard, the other patrons being surprised, and your having to return later, embarrassed, with the bib and your payment for the unfinished cut? Even if they are unlikely to occur, you will need to embrace the possibility of these negative events, because you won't necessarily be able to shake them out of your mind. The next best thing is to be willing to go through them.

Listen: it is not simply that you need to put up with such embarrassments. The irony is that when you *do* change your mind— when you are *willing* to go through such struggles—that new stance will reduce the likelihood of such events occurring. So, it is worth the investment to learn this skill.

And how could you handle such embarrassments? First, you must become one hundred percent committed to getting better, so committed that you will do whatever it takes to get control of your life. Second, you need to recognize that panic thrives on what we call "thoughts of impending doom." Panic makes its living on scaring you with catastrophic predictions. It wins when you respond to those catastrophic fantasies with: A) "Oh, no, that could really happen!" and B) "I can't tolerate that. It would be horrible if that happened."

And, third, you have to decide that you will cope with whatever happens. If you feel embarrassed at the party, you decide to handle your embarrassment. If the person you were talking to had a contact for a new job you were interested in and now probably won't recommend you, you choose to tolerate that loss. Perhaps you are really strapped for money and that job would have been a real shot-in-the-arm. Not getting the recommendation may be a blow to your financial situation. Willingly choose to handle that, too. Why? Because if you perceive that you can cope with a negative event, then you will be willing to enter that event. Avoidance out of fear and threat is what keeps you stuck. Support your efforts to push into threatening circumstances by believing you will figure out a way to cope with whatever happens.

Panic wants you to think, "I can't tolerate that consequence." The degree you allow yourself to cope with any negative event is the degree that you grab control away from panic. Get to the place where you can say, "Come on, panic, give me your best shot. I can handle it." What exactly do you need to handle? Four experiences: your physical sensations, your emotional response, missed opportunities, and the judgments of others.

- *Your physical sensations.* Anxiety is uncomfortable. If my heart started racing or I became dizzy, I would instantly be scared (which, of course, would set off my Emergency Response, causing my racing heart and my dizziness to get even stronger). But you also know now that these sensations are not dangerous; therefore, you can learn to handle them. To overcome panic, you need to practice tolerating your uncomfortable sensations. Purposely, voluntarily choose to get anxious and sit with those sensations. Then you can tell yourself, "I can handle this," and you will believe your words. When you willingly experience uncomfortable sensations, you can't be blackmailed by them.
- *Your emotional response.* Being embarrassed, self-conscious, self-critical, humiliated, disappointed, sad, frustrated, ashamed—these are all familiar feelings for people with panic. No matter how much you want to support and love yourself, you are going to get tangled up in psychologically uncomfortable responses to having a panic attack or escaping an event out of fear or performing poorly because of anxiety. Most people want to avoid these feelings, but that isn't your smartest strategy.

Your best course is to take care of your uncomfortable reactions instead of trying to banish them.

When you imagine the possibility of abruptly leaving that conversation at the party and feeling embarrassed later, then develop your ability to say and *believe,* "That could happen, and if I feel embarrassed, I won't like that, but I can cope with it. I want to get better badly enough that I am willing to be embarrassed. I will find a way to handle it."

How do you learn to tolerate being embarrassed?

1. Know that you have to tolerate being embarrassed. It comes with the territory of getting better. You gotta do what you gotta do.
2. You don't need to feel embarrassed with one hundred percent of your consciousness. You are more than just timid and fearful. There is a part of you who cares for you when you act courageously. Find ways to support yourself. "This is absolutely hard. And I'm really uncomfortable. But I know I can get stronger. This is the key through that door. I can stick with it." If you need help in this area, I'll be teaching you more about this inner voice—which I call your Supportive Observer—in Chapter 17. Your Supportive Observer will help carry you through.
3. Turn to supportive people who will remind you what important work you are doing in your healing process.
4. Put yourself in situations where you can generate awkwardness or embarrassment. Do what you are afraid to do. Then practice taking care of yourself. That's how you will learn that you can cope.

Are you sensing a theme here? If you believe you cannot tolerate an experience, you will avoid it. That's why you are stuck now. When you learn to cope with an experience—whether it is anxiety, embarrassment or an event that didn't go according to your plan—then you will be less intimidated and more willing to move forward into it.

- *Missed opportunities.* If you decide to go to a movie even though you tend to get anxious in theaters, then you may not be able to concentrate on or enjoy that movie. If you choose to have lunch alone at a restaurant even though that often provokes your anxiety, then you may not get much pleasure from that meal. You might not even feel hungry. If you commit yourself to take a commercial flight in two weeks, even though you get anxious during turbulence, then it's possible you might have some days beforehand when you don't concentrate as well on your tasks. You could have some nights during those two weeks in which you don't sleep that well.

To overcome the dominance of anxiety in your life, you need to be willing to sacrifice your concentration, sleep, performance, and enjoyment. These will be temporary sacrifices, but they will be hardships nonetheless. How badly do you want to get better? Badly enough to make these sacrifices? Then you are developing the right attitude.

- *Judgments of others.* This one can be tough to embrace. Who wants anyone to see them anxiously pull off the highway when driving, or fumble for words in a conversation, or leave in the middle of an appointment? Yet the most powerful position to take as you consider these events is to be willing to tolerate the judgments of others and the emotions you may have in response to those judgments.

Some people choose to be self-revealing about their problems, supporting their efforts to move forward while risking the criticisms of others.

Brian has worked with me three different times over the past decade, and he was quite dedicated in his efforts, since his family lived more than an hour away from my office. When he first came to see me as a sixteen-year-old, his panic attacks included times when he was standing on the pitcher's mound for his high school baseball team. What courage! Occasionally as he readied himself for a pitch, panic would come rushing in. And he would handle it. He'd take a calming breath, wait for 15 to 20 seconds while he focused his attention again, and throw his next pitch. We worked on fine-tuning his strategy in those moments, but he was doing pretty well on his own. One of his biggest advantages was that his coach knew about his panic disorder and supported his efforts. And he was a damn good pitcher.

I saw him two years later as panic returned while he was away at a distant college. Once again, Brian impressed me with his forthrightness. For instance, if he were eating dinner over the holidays with his parents and their guests, he would typically begin the meal telling the visitors about his situation. "I just want you to know that sometimes I have panic attacks when I'm at the dinner table. I'm fine, but you might notice an expression on my face, or I might need to get up and leave the room for a few minutes. I hope that's OK with you." Now sometimes that embarrassed Brian's parents. But it is one of the primary reasons he has been so successful at mastering his panic: he refuses to be blackmailed by shame and embarrassment.

"I Want This"

I've been talking about changing your position of "I must stay on guard against anxiety" to one of "I can drop my guard," and shifting the belief of "I can't tolerate this" to one of "I can handle this." There is a third message that is equally powerful: "I want this." What will this stance give you? Here's an explanation you might use. In an anxious moment you won't be doing this much mental talking. But this is the logic behind the simple message of, "I want this."

> Oh, yikes! I didn't expect to get anxious here. This is a surprise. I'm scared about how bad my feelings are going to get. But this is good, because I need to be practicing my new attitude of "I want this" by facing anxiety head-on every day. And here it is! So I'm going to welcome it. Resisting my fear is going to increase my fear. If I fight it or keep trying to get rid of it, then I'm doing exactly what panic expects: I'll be labeling it as dangerous, I'll become more anxious, and I'll feel out of control. So I'm going to hang out here, breathe into my anxiety, do the best I can to concentrate on my task, and see what happens. These feelings are definitely uncomfortable, but I expect that, and I can handle them.
>
> What if it gets worse! Well, if that happens, then I'll handle that, too. But one step at a time. A racing heart and dizziness is what I'm feeling *now,* and I want this feeling.

Listen carefully: You are *not* taking this stance to reduce your anxiety or panic. This is *not* a ploy to avoid feeling anxious. It is to reflect your choice to join with your anxiety instead of fight with it. It requires you to be courageous, because you are not yet certain about the results. You choose to embrace your discomfort and your doubt. You have faith that you can handle whatever happens. By doing so you become powerful.

People are not powerful by imposing their will on the world, even though our society gives such people status. You will become powerful when you accept that life can change your most cherished plans. If that happens, then create new plans in light of your new experience. You will become powerful in a threatening situation by accepting your fear. Incorporate it into your acceptable sense of self. And whatever realistic predictions you make about possible trouble, believe that you can cope with them. This is the formula that will teach your body-&-mind to turn off the alarm.

Frequent, Intense, and Long

The cardinal rules in behavior therapy for phobias have been in place for over thirty years, and they are highly successful. Every behavior therapist I know in the world (and I know a lot) agrees with these principles—the principles of habituation. To recover from a phobia and to have confidence that you are over it, you need to combine three experiences in your treatment:

1. Frequency: You must face the threat repeatedly over several weeks.
2. Intensity: Your body-&-mind need to wrestle with whatever strong sensations of fear you might have. Muting or avoiding those sensations will slow your progress.
3. Duration: It is important to face the threat long enough for your body-&-mind to learn to manage it.

Then and only then will you discover that you can handle the irrational fears of that phobia.

Now—just so you know—I am not a behavior therapist. I am a cognitive therapist. I help people with anxiety change their beliefs, and that's what I'm going to do with you. These three habituation principles will be immensely helpful to us, and they are going to play a central role in our project. However, I think our approach of influencing your beliefs will speed up your process of change and will stabilize any gains you make with habituation.

So let's continue that conversation in your mind, adding in these three valuable guidelines. Again, you won't really be saying this in the distressing moment; the guidelines are the justifications for saying "I want this" when you face anxiety and uncertainty.

> I actually know how to get better, because I know what the research has proven. To handle a threatening experience, I want to do three things. First, I want to step into that uncomfortable situation *frequently*. My impulse is to avoid in order to stay comfortable and in control. But I want to become uncomfortable and not sure of my control so I can win this game. I want to do that over and over again. If I don't face this stuff often enough, I won't get strong. So, good, here I am practicing being uncomfortable and uncertain.

Choose to voluntarily, purposely become uncomfortable and unsure of your control. Why? Because that is what currently scares you. Go *toward* what scares you to conquer it. Listen to what First Lady Eleanor Roosevelt once said: "You have to learn to face what scares you. You gain strength, courage and confidence by every experience in which you really stop to look fear in the face. You are able to say to yourself, 'I have lived through this horror. I can take the next thing that comes along.' You must do the thing you think you cannot do."

It isn't just that you need to feel uncomfortable and unsure. You've probably experienced that plenty of times. The goal is to purposely, voluntarily choose to be uncomfortable and uncertain. This is an attitude shift, not just a shift in behavior. Why take that stance of "purposely, voluntarily choosing"? Because that is the best strategy for *reducing* your discomfort. Here's more of your mental conversation.

This is the second action I want to take to handle my sense of threat: it's clear by the research that I need to be distressed enough when I practice. If I just go into situations where I can generate some anxiety, but not much, then my body-&-mind won't learn what it needs to learn. I want to be pretty darn uncomfortable. On a scale of '0' to '100', I want to get up to at least a '50'; that's how to get better. I want to get better. I want to get better in the long run more than I want to stay comfortable at this moment. I do look forward to being in this same situation in the future and feeling comfortable. I'll get there by being uncomfortable now. So . . . great! I'm uncomfortable. This is what I want. I don't feel very good, and I can handle that.

You don't need to dive into high anxiety situations right now. A great start is to put yourself into low level threat situations that allow you to practice saying and believing, "I can handle this, and I want this." Listen in to another way you might convince yourself to want the discomfort you are feeling.

Here is the other thing that the research is clear about: People who overcome panic are people who practice staying in threatening situations—while they are at least moderately uncomfortable—*for a long time*. Often they shoot for staying there for 45 to 90 minutes. The body-&-mind needs to learn to tolerate that environment, and that takes time lingering in that location, while staying at least moderately distressed.

Geez, I'm uncomfortable! I can handle it, but this is hard! I sure hope it helps in the long run, because I'm not having a very pleasant feeling. But it's great that I'm here, and I'm glad my anxiety is this strong. Because this is how I get better. I only hope it can stick around for a while, because I really want this practice to count.

You don't need to start by staying for long periods of time in all your threatening situations. But do work on the task of choosing to experience exactly what you have been avoiding. This is a profound attitude shift. How do you apply this attitude to the fears you have? Begin by deciding to practice a new stance:

> I'm going to drop my guard against anxiety. I can handle being anxious, and I want to get anxious.

There is a synergy at play here. You need to discover that you can handle anxiety before you can believe your statement, "I want to get anxious." As you face anxiety with the message, "I want this," then you will discover that this attitude literally helps you handle your anxiety. Don't go looking for that result. When you require "positive" results, you are resisting the moment. So practice without expectation and find out what you notice over time.

"It's OK That I'm Anxious Right Now"

Thinking out loud with Camille a dozen years ago helped me put a bigger piece of the puzzle together.

Camille N. called me from Florida. She suffered from panic attacks and recently found a copy of *Don't Panic* in the library. She was wondering if, on her trip back to New York, she could stop in for a consultation. We set up the appointment, and Camille arrived as scheduled.

Camille turned out to be a dedicated student of self-help techniques. She practiced formal relaxation daily. She was very experienced in her breathing skills. She generated practice sessions in anxiety-provoking situations and knew the most supportive self-talk during panicky times. But she kept having trouble.

> Like last week, for instance. I was driving down the boulevard at about four-thirty, and the traffic was moderate. I needed to take a left, so at the stop light I moved over

into the turn lane, three lanes from the right curb and pulled up behind four cars. Immediately three more cars pulled in behind me and the other two lanes filled with traffic. These lights are notoriously slow, and I've always hated getting trapped like that.

When I felt my stomach get tense, I knew I had to work with my skills. First I reassured myself that I could handle this. If I needed to, I could even get out of the car, leave it right there at the light. I took a nice big Calming Breath, then started Natural Breathing. I dropped my hands from the steering wheel and let them relax in my lap. Nothing seemed to help!

Outwardly I was attentive and positive, but inwardly I was frustrated, thinking, "Why? Why wasn't that helping? That should be working!" I felt like the Wizard of Oz. This woman has driven so far in anticipation of this specifically arranged meeting with the expert who wrote the book she depends on to get well. Now here we are, face to face, and I'm about to say, "Hmm, I'm not sure what else to suggest."

I'd love to be able to say, "Then it dawned on me . . ." In reality it took another thirty minutes of struggle to see the new opening. Both Camille and I were making the same error, and you can hear it in our self-talk. She says, "Nothing seemed to help!" I said to myself, "Why wasn't that helping? That should be working!"

Despite all our combined years of study, we were unknowingly committing a basic mistake. Our immediate goal was for Camille to stop feeling anxious. We thought if she applied enough technique—handle your negative talk, get your breathing straight, be willing to tolerate symptoms, wait—she would get results of diminished anxiety. "What's wrong with that?" you say?

Here's the answer, which may be tough to accept. While the long-term goal is to diminish your anxiety, the immediate goal is to continually monitor your attitude—*to accept exactly what you are experiencing, as you experience it.* As soon as you say, "This had better work," you are moving against this important task. It is fine to observe, study, and learn from your current experience, but don't declare that your feelings must change on demand. Our body-&-mind simply doesn't work that way.

This is paradox in its purest form. The attitude to aim for is, "It's OK that I'm anxious right now." You might simultaneously fool around with getting rid of the anxiety. You can try every trick and gimmick you know, apply all your concentration, tenacity, and commitment to the task of reducing the anxiety. If you take that tack, then you must also hold this attitude: "If it works, that'll be great. And if it doesn't work—if I'm still anxious— *that'll be OK, too.*"

This is the attitude that even the best students of panic tend to miss. You must step up onto the platform of acceptance. Apply your skills from there. Maintain that stance through all the good and bad responses you get to your skills. And end up standing there in the end—accepting exactly what you are experiencing—regardless of the outcome.

Attitude as Technique

The most important point here is that this position—"It's OK that I'm anxious right now"—is not about passive resignation to the status quo. It is not surrendering to the fact that "you have panic attacks and you better get used to it." Instead, it is part of an active, dynamic process of healing. Think of this attitude as a technique that you apply throughout the moments you are either anticipating or having trouble. When you say, "This had better work," you are testing yourself and you will respond by emotionally and physically tightening up. When you tighten up, you feed panic. By saying, "It's OK if it doesn't work," you pull yourself out of this testing environment. Crazy as it sounds, this action of removing the demand for success actually increases the likelihood of your success.

Someone once said that if you want to hit the bull's-eye every time, throw the dart first and then draw the circles around it. There will be plenty of hardships coming your way before the final curtain. You might as well get on friendly terms with them. Say yes to them when they arrive. Then begin to manipulate them actively and creatively. The fear of being trapped is a common concern for people with panic. Freedom comes by saying yes to whatever trap life puts you in, then doing something to get yourself out. Whenever one of your attempts fails, begin immediately to do the really hard work: accept that you are still stuck in discomfort. Take time to complete that task of accepting the dissatisfying outcome first. Then redouble your efforts to change that outcome next time.

Your Worried Thoughts

When you face anxiety and uncertainty, there is no way that you will be saying "I want this" with all your heart, mind, and soul. There will be a solid, still powerful part of you that will be saying,

> Are you nuts!?! No, I don't want this feeling! I don't want it to last or get stronger. That's ridiculous! I'm scared. What if I get so confused right now that I can't perform? What if my heart races so much that I have a full-blown panic attack? I need to do some relaxation to get rid of this feeling. Or, better yet, let me step outside and calm down.

That's why I am saying that you will need all the courage you can conjure up. "I want this" will have plenty of competition, and that competition will stem from your sense that you are protecting yourself from danger. Your worried thoughts will be a powerful competing force coming from deep within you.

- *Expect to hear that voice.* Account for it. Know it is running side by side with this new little voice inside you trying to say, "I want this, and I can handle this." How should you respond to a commanding message of threat such as, "This will be terrifying"? Mentally step back from it, hear it, and want it too. That's what fear sounds like. And it is the most important element of your anxiety that you will need to manage. You should want it because it is already there. You can hear it make its presence known in your mind. Don't resist something that is already present in your life; that will only promote your suffering. When you hear that inner frightened voice saying, "This is terrifying. I can't do this!," then focus your attention on supporting yourself. "It's fine I just had that thought. I'm supposed to, because I'm feeling threatened here." That doesn't mean that you must *act* on your worried thought and run out of the event. Know it for what it is: the part of you that is scared. It exists in all of us, and it has a right to exist inside any of us. You just don't want it to be the dominant, prevailing voice.

Face a threat while hearing yourself *voice* the threat. That's how you get control back. Don't try to quiet your negative thoughts. Simply notice them, refrain from allowing them to dictate your next actions, and linger in the situation a while longer.

Moving Forward

These attitudes are not simply philosophical underpinnings. They are active workhorses in your healing process. Think of attitudes in a new way; think of them as technique.

- I'll become stronger by purposely facing what I am afraid of.

- It's OK that I'm anxious right now.
- I can handle these sensations.
- I can handle this uncertainty.
- I want this anxiety.
- I want this uncertainty.
- Love the mat.
- Run toward the roar.

To find the benefits for you, don't wait until you are having a panic attack. Write these statements on an index card and carry them with you throughout the day. Pull them out when you're feeling uncomfortable and stuck. Use them to influence what you do (or don't do) next. That's a good way to learn of their benefits. It is also consistent with the metaphor of inoculation: You start by learning to accept a small amount of discomfort and build your confidence on that experience. Nobody learns to drive by entering the Indianapolis 500. A much easier place to begin is the mall parking lot on Sunday morning, with your supportive parent sitting next to you. Master these attitudes by giving them a chance in lower-risk situations. Then gradually turn your attention to those panic-provoking situations.

Who knows? Maybe these are the only "techniques" you'll need.

CHAPTER 11

Experience:
The Greatest Teacher

Most people try to handle panic by managing their uncomfortable sensations whenever they appear. That's an understandable approach, but an insufficient one. In Chapter 10 you learned that the most effective way to win over panic is to *seek it out,* to run toward the roar. All the new knowledge and skills regarding anxiety attacks that you have gathered so far prepare you for the important job of *approaching* the situations that you fear.

Looking for Trouble

Here is the best way to begin: be proactive, not reactive. Don't wait for anxiety-provoking situations to arrive; look around your world for ways to stir up trouble. Ask yourself, "What can I do to get myself anxious today?" Don't concern yourself with how to get strong anxiety or doubt (that's a relief, eh?) or how to get it to last. Simply work on this one attitude: wanting it.

Look for conditions in which you are willing to say, "I want this." If you end up in a situation that you perceive to be too threatening, don't expect to practice there. Back up to situations that are less threatening. You can begin simply by thinking of entering an anxiety-provoking situation. But you have to think about it realistically enough to feel anxiety. If you can't provoke any anxiety that way, then put yourself in a location where you can generate low-grade distress, perhaps one that you can escape from easily or one that only lasts a short time. For example, if restaurants are too threatening for you right now, drive to a restaurant, sit in your car in their parking lot and imagine yourself walking in. As you get anxious in response to that image practice saying and believing, "I want this feeling." (Why do you want it? Because you want to get better, and learning to want the discomfort is your most important building block to getting better.) Then just sit with your feelings of discomfort without trying to "fix" them.

Everywhere you go, anything you do, look for opportunities to embrace your discomfort. Literally say it in your mind—"I want this." Work on *believing* that message. Why believe it?

- Because wanting is the opposite of resisting, and resisting makes anxiety worse.
- Because wanting is the opposite of avoiding, and avoiding makes fear more powerful.
- Because wanting is the opposite of what panic expects you to say, and that screws with panic's head.

To accept your discomfort and doubt is important. The message, "It's OK that I'm anxious here," reflects your belief that you can handle these feelings. Acceptance is important. However, this is a step beyond acceptance. I am encouraging you to add a more deliberate, powerful message of "I want this." Remember the principles of habituation that I outlined in the last chapter. Your ultimate goal is to voluntarily, purposefully seek out the three components of habituation:

- frequent encounters with events
- that allow you to generate at least moderate distress and uncertainty
- while you remain in those events for an extended length of time

As you begin, your task is to taste what that experience is like by practicing during relatively low-threat events or by anticipating the possibility of a threatening experience prior to entering an event.

Here are some examples of how you might practice this skill. (These are merely illustrations, not instructions.) Imagine that you are someone bothered by each of these settings.

. . .

You are about to give your report at the weekly departmental meeting and you can feel your heart racing. You hear yourself say, "Geez, I hope people don't pick up on the nervousness in my voice." Tell yourself, "I want this nervousness. And I can handle the possibility that people will notice." Clear your mind of other thoughts for a minute or two and simply allow yourself to be anxious. After that minute or two do whatever else you want to do or typically do. But introduce this strategy into the mix for a bit. Remember: Give yourself the message, and then sit with the experience before you rush off to get rid of the feelings.

. . .

You are standing in line at the bank and your legs feel weak while your head seems to swim. Listen in on whatever your negative thoughts are, like, "I'm getting worse by the second! I can't stand here any longer; I've got to get out of here." Accept those fearful thoughts without acting on them. After all, that's exactly what it's supposed to sound like in our minds when we're facing our fears: we don't think we can take it, and we want it to end. Then tell yourself, "I *want* these weak legs. I *want* this dizziness. Tolerating these sensations is good practice. This doesn't mean that I'll collapse. But even if I do, I'll handle it." If you feel so scared that you immediately get out of line and leave the bank, tell yourself, "I was looking for that kind of scary experience, and I got a little taste of it. Good. I want to touch on that again later." Take a break for a half hour if you need to. Then see if you can practice another standing-in-line-and-feeling-uncomfortable experience. *Want* that.

. . .

Your daughter has just finished soccer practice. You are crossing the field to meet her, and suddenly you feel overwhelmed and disoriented by the open space. Practice saying, "I can handle this. I want this." Do whatever you can to linger with that sensation. This is *practice*. You need to practice to get stronger, and you certainly want to get stronger. Even if you stop crossing the field and walk around the periphery instead, first give yourself a few moments to experience and welcome the discomfort. While you are backing away from the threat of the open field, you will still have residual feelings of discomfort. Practice wanting them and reminding yourself that you can cope with them, even though you know they are about to subside. Welcome your discomfort, even as it is fading.

In any of these situations, even if you are withdrawing or using a crutch to reduce your discomfort, continue to embrace the message of, "I can handle this. I want this."

While you are practicing, you might have an insight. Your awareness could come in the form of, "Hey! I was just sitting there, trying to practice 'I can handle this; I want this' when I noticed that my anxiety actually reached a plateau and flattened off. That's interesting." During another practice your aha! moment might be, "Hey! Once I said 'I want this' and I just lingered there without escaping, my anxiety decreased. That's a surprise."

To give yourself the chance to have a new learning in an old troubling scene you will have to be courageous. Keep in mind that you are combating the belief of, "I need to stop this doubt and discomfort." The definition of courage is to be scared and do it anyway. That is absolutely what you will be doing in the face of threat: you will be standing there and taking it. There is no way you can accomplish this goal of "I can handle this; I want this" unless you are scared.

Here is a paradox for you. *Don't* practice to get those revelations. Practice simply to practice, without regard to the results. The absolutely best way to work on these skills is to not expect any particular outcome. Practice, practice, practice, without expectation. Trust that practice will lead you to awareness, and awareness will propel you into facing other threatening situations.

Prepare for Your Practice

Let's begin by focusing on that question, "What can I do to get myself anxious today?" Actually, we'll work on identifying opportunities to practice in the next two days, identifying what you might worry about, assessing how realistic those feared consequences are, and deciding how you will cope with each of them.

Identify opportunities to feel anxious and worried. Think about the activities you have planned only for today and tomorrow. As you imagine entering each event, look for chances to say "yes" to any of these questions:

- Can I create some anxiety here?
- Can I practice being willing to be anxious here?

- Can I generate some doubt about how things will turn out?
- Can I explore tolerating that sense of "not knowing" in this situation?

Use the form below to briefly describe activities in the next two days that fit as "yes" events.

Form 1: Opportunities to Practice Your Skills	
Choose to Feel Anxious—Choose to Feel Uncertain	
Today	Tomorrow

If you generate very few items, that may reflect how you have kept yourself safe by avoiding discomfort. That's certainly understandable, but it's time to venture out. Ask yourself, "What could I add to the day to generate some anxiety and doubt?" You need to engage in activities to create opportunities.

Identify what you worry about. In each situation, list the specific consequences that scare you, using Form 2 on page 209. (You'll be using a new Form 2 for each event. You can freely download a copy of all these forms at www.dontpaniclive.com so that you can use them again in the future.) For example, imagine that you are anticipating having trouble when you have to give a report at your office. You might have several fears:

"People will hear nervousness in my voice."
"I won't be very articulate because I'll be so nervous."
"I'll be fired for incompetence."

How realistic is that possibility? Some of the threats you list may be likely, but others might be exaggerated and improbable. Can you tell the difference? Help yourself out by rating the likelihood of each consequence in that second column of Form 2. Think of the rating as a continuum from "highly unlikely" to "highly likely." If you are thinking about your departmental report, what is your opinion of the likelihood of people hearing your voice tremble? On a 0–10 scale, you might appraise it as a "7."

People will hear nervousness in my voice.

```
    0----------------------5-------X----------------------10
    Highly unlikely          Possible          Highly likely
```

However, when you think about your worry of "I'll be fired for incompetence," perhaps you are able to downgrade the risk of this happening. Maybe you tell yourself, "Yes, it would be awful if I got fired over this, but that's not a worry I need to focus on." That outcome might rate a "2."

I'll be fired for incompetence.

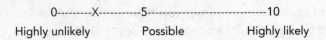

```
    0---------X-----------5------------------------------10
    Highly unlikely          Possible          Highly likely
```

If you are worried about an outcome that is highly unlikely, then diminish its importance, even if only to a small degree. If you really want to perform the task on your list, why allow your mind to float over to the worst-case outcome? By focusing your attention away from the extremely unlikely events, you can better concentrate on the task at hand.

Form 2: Coping with Specific Fears		
Event:		
Feared Consequences	Likelihood (0–10)	How I'll Cope If It Occurs

Know how you will tolerate any consequences. Decide which of your many skills, points of view, actions, and resources can assist you in tolerating every single one of your feared consequences listed in the first column and add them to the third column of Form 2. If you fear the consequence of "I won't be very articulate," maybe you'll choose to "clarify my main talking points on a handout" as a backup. By listing all your feared consequences and how you'll handle them, the ultimate goal is to be able to think, "Whatever happens in this situation, I'll handle it." Over time, you may find that on a number of items you simply write, "I'll handle it somehow." That's an excellent response! Then you won't be allowing your intimidation to stop you.

If you fail to create a coping strategy for even one of the threatening consequences, then your mind will tend to gravitate to that fear. For example, suppose you decide, "If I get anxious, that's OK. If I feel a little light-headed, I can cope with that and keep going. But I hope I don't have a full-blown panic attack. That would be awful, and I don't know how I'll handle the humiliation." That threat of getting panicky will cause you to feel far more anxious and worried than is necessary and will limit your ability to concentrate on the activity. Come up with a way to tolerate it all, including the possibility of a panic attack. In this scenario, perhaps you will say, "If I have a full-blown panic attack, I'll excuse myself and leave the room. I'll definitely feel embarrassed, but I'll deal with that. I'll just tell them I was feeling physically sick."

Be willing to handle anything. Here is another paradoxical move: No matter how unlikely the consequence, if you are still worried that it is a possible outcome, then you need to be willing to tolerate it. There is no other way to win this game. Telling yourself, "It's highly unlikely that I'll be fired," won't remove that fear from your consciousness. A strong response to this fear is, "It's highly unlikely that I'll get fired for this, and I really don't see any benefit in dwelling on that fear. But if I were to get fired, then I'll recover from that, too. It'll pose problems, but I'll get through them. I want to get better badly enough that I am willing to tolerate the ever-so-slight possibility of losing my job."

You don't have much choice about this matter of risk-taking; it comes with the territory. People with anxiety tend to want a one hundred percent guarantee that nothing is going to go wrong. If there is the slightest risk of a serious problem, they want to remove that risk. Even if there's a slim chance you could be fired, your tendency will be to worry about it.

Even if you have never fainted while standing in a line at the bank or walking across an open field, if you worry that there is a slight chance of it, you will feel threatened by it. Therefore, you must believe that you will figure out how to cope with even the most unlikely, worst outcomes. Fainting at the bank? It's highly unlikely that you will. But if you do? Someone will call 911, and as you gain consciousness, the paramedics will appraise whether you need to be transported to the emergency room. Perhaps you will bump your head. And you'll probably feel embarrassed. If you are currently afraid of fainting while standing in line at the bank, then you need to trust that you can handle even that dramatic event. You might be sore and you might feel embarrassed, and it may cost you three hundred dollars to get transported to the ER. But you will survive! You have to want to get over your anxiety problem badly enough to be willing to tolerate all that. Then you will start taking control of panic.

On Form 2, I'm asking you to state how you will cope. While doing this exercise you will begin to realize that you can handle these threats if they arise. Once you get the hang of it, then there won't be a need for you to know specifically how you will cope with each possibility, as long as you believe, "I'll handle it somehow."

Once you have identified your opportunities to practice in the next two days and you have developed your coping responses to each of the consequences, use them to help you decide which activities you will approach.

Begin Your Practice

Based on your answers on Form 2, which events are you willing to use to practice your skills? For those events, consider practicing in two phases: anticipating an event and then entering that event. Each phase can stand alone as a positive practice experience. Working only with Stage 1, you don't have to *enter* any of these situations; you can simply practice approaching them. Whether it is speaking up at a meeting, standing in line, or crossing an open field, you may practice approaching a situation six or seven times and purposely never enter it, as a way to build up your skill of wanting distress and uncertainty.

PRACTICE YOUR SKILLS

STAGE 1: *Purposely Anticipate Events*

Before you enter into any threatening event, start practicing.

1. *Imagine entering the event and purposely let your anticipation generate some anxiety and doubt.*
2. *As you notice your anxiety, practice accepting and wanting those feelings.* "OK, I'm imagining myself standing

in line at the bank, and now I'm anxious. Really anxious! Yikes, this is scary! But . . . good. I want this. Right this second I am practicing. This counts!"

3. *Linger with your anxiety.* Don't be in a rush to escape the feeling. Hang out with your distress. Give your body-&-mind time to respond to your message of, "I can handle this anxiety, and I want this."

4. *Listen in on your worries and remind yourself that you can cope with whatever happens. Then practice wanting those worried thoughts as well as the anxiety.* When you hear yourself say, "I'm dizzy; I could faint!" say something like, "That's a good, anxiety-provoking thought. I want that thought, too." Don't do anything with the thought. Don't embellish it or encourage it. Don't talk yourself out of it. Notice it and accept it as an expected fearful thought in such a situation. Then wait for the next threatening thought or feeling.

5. *If you get quiet and relaxed, return to Step 1.* Introduce distress again, so you'll have something to practice.

Keep repeating this practice as many times as you need until you can tolerate the anxiety you purposely generate. Once you can say to yourself, "When this type of anxiety and doubt rise up, I can handle it," then you are ready to take your practice to the next level. Move to Stage 2, where you will step into the threatening situation with those same skills.

But first I want to give you a pep talk. . . .

This Is Not a Test

I hope that I will never take another exam to receive another certification within my profession. Even though, at fifty-seven, I still consider myself a perpetual student in this field, I'm no longer interested in jumping through hoops to prove to someone else that I can do my job as a psychologist.

The last exam I took was to become a licensed psychologist. I can remember what it was like preparing: four months of studying fifteen hours per week, plus holding down a job. If I failed the exam, I'd have to take it again in six months, and eventually I'd have to pass it to be a psychologist. I worried going in because in Massachusetts, where I lived at the time, only a certain percentage of psychologists can pass; many people must fail each test, not on the basis of their score, but on the ranking of their score. I passed that exam. But during the months, days, and especially hours before it, I had to work on handling my worry as well as my knowledge areas.

In Stage 2 of "Practice Your Skills" you will practice some tasks that are quite new to you. You may feel awkward, clumsy, confused, and quite unskilled. You need to support all your efforts, even if you aren't instantly getting the results you expect. However, it seems that people who are prone to panic attacks turn many experiences into tests. When you decide to enter a previously difficult situation, do you say, "This will be a test of how well I can cope"? As soon as you declare it a test, your body is going to secrete adrenaline, because you will be saying to yourself, "Uh-oh. I'd better do well," while you simultaneously imagine yourself failing. That process will cause you to feel anxious. The more you set up future events as tests, the more you are going to feel anxious.

People declare, "This is a test" before an event, and they declare, "I failed that test" after the event. I have watched clients improve steadily week after week. Then, one week, they inevitably have a small setback in their progress. From this one episode they become dejected, depressed, and demoralized. They are full of self-critical and hopeless thoughts. They don't simply say, "I failed." They follow it with "and I shouldn't have," or "and that means I should quit trying," or "What's the point?" or "That proves I'll never change."

As you begin taking action, your attitude about the task will be an important factor in your progress. Consider any activity you engage in as *practice*. Never view a future task as a *test* of your progress or of your ability to overcome panic. And don't look back at an attempted task to label your efforts a failure. In other words, don't invest your sense of self-worth in the positive or negative outcome of your plans. Put your self-worth in your willingness to expend effort in approaching instead of avoiding.

When you decide that all your experiences are practice, you are in effect saying that you are both willing and able to learn from each experience. You might fail to meet a certain goal by a specific time, but your intentions aren't a failure, and your efforts aren't a failure. They are the successful ways that people learn: setting goals and applying effort. No one knows everything about any particular subject. Our greatest scientists continually create new questions to ask about their fields of expertise. These brilliant men and women would be the first to defend the importance of maintaining the open, curious, exploratory mind of a student.

When you test yourself during any activity, you inhibit your learning. If you say to yourself, "That action I took yesterday proves that I'm never going to make it," you essentially have said, "I shouldn't bother learning from yesterday; it's too late for me." Of course, the truth of the matter is that making mistakes and studying them are among our best learning tools.

Since *everyone* who takes on challenges has setbacks, you can assume you will, too. When you hear your self-critical or hopeless comments rise up, let them go. They are just noise, and they will distract you from learning.

It's true that if you set a target of remaining at a party until eleven P.M., but your discomfort causes you to leave at nine-thirty, then you failed to meet your goal. That is like throwing a dart at the bull's-eye and missing it by three rings. Let that experience be feedback to you as you take corrective action. What can you adjust for your next throw? Can you take aim at a different spot on the target? Give the dart more arc on the throw? Concentrate on your follow-through? Step closer to the target?

As you approach these first events by following the guidelines of Stage 2, concentrate on what you can do to improve your outcome. If you leave a scene without meeting your goal, there are two important focal points for your attention. The first is, "What can I learn from my experience in that situation that I can apply next time?" The second is, "How can I take care of myself now that I am leaving this difficult situation?" Practice the skill of supporting yourself while facing a disappointment. If your goal is improving your performance next time, how do you want to treat yourself after your difficulty this time? Stop being critical of yourself and begin developing a supportive voice within you.

Let's begin Stage 2.

PRACTICE YOUR SKILLS

STAGE 2: *Purposely Enter Events*

1. *As you enter, and while you are in the scene, focus your attention on your task.* If you're performing a simple task, such as standing in line at the bank, then you can attend to any simple thing you want, such as what you see around you. If you are engaged in a more complex skill, such as giving a report in a departmental meeting, focus on your skills, such as delivering your content and responding to the requests of those listening.

2. *Practice accepting and wanting any anxiety that you notice.* Remind yourself that you are looking for frequency, intensity, and duration of distress.

3. *Linger in the moment of being anxious and uncertain.* Give your body-&-mind time to respond to your message of, "I can handle this, and I want this." Don't be in a rush to escape your feelings; hang out with your distress. And don't get derailed by your negative thoughts. Notice them, accept and want them, allow

them to hang around, but don't bother reacting to
them. Then refocus on your task.

4. *Remind yourself that you can cope with whatever happens.*

Practice, Practice, Practice

Take these principles into your world today and tomorrow and
work on them. Repetition is the key, so practice as often as you
can. Several times daily would be great. Each new day, use
Forms 1 and 2 to generate new opportunities to practice and
learn. Set as your goal to practice these attitude skills until you
believe in their benefits and you are successful in applying them
to your threatening situations. Don't quickly evaluate how you
are doing and decide you can't be successful. Just work the program, again and again.

Remember that you win over panic by not resisting. Be patient and you will eventually get a spontaneous insight. It might
sound like this: "Hey! Four out of the last twelve times when I
said, 'I can handle this; I want this,' and really meant it, my
anxiety just faded away. Another five times I stayed anxious, but
I handled it fine. It didn't leave, and I didn't freak out. Maybe it
really is all about how I respond. Cool."

When to Move to the Next Skills

You will be ready for the next phase of your practice when you
can say "yes" to each statement in the following list:

How Do You Know You Are Succeeding?

☐ You look for opportunities to provoke your anxiety
and distress.
☐ You can figure out what specific consequences you are
afraid of.

☐ You challenge your tendency to focus on unrealistic consequences.

☐ You can think of ways that you can cope with those consequences, whether realistic or unrealistic, if they occur.

☐ You purposely choose to feel uncomfortable and uncertain within your threatening situations: "I want this."

☐ You choose to linger with your anxiety and uncertainty instead of escaping.

☐ You notice your negative and fearful thoughts without getting caught up in them. You accept them without getting rid of them.

When to switch to Part IV, Support When You Need It: If you cannot get to this attitude shift in any of your fearful situations, even after three practices a day for two weeks, then switch to Part IV, which begins with Chapter 15. That program will strengthen your skills so that you can return here later to continue this work.

CHAPTER 12

Look for More

D o you remember playing checkers as a child, near the end of the game, when you have one piece left and the other kid has four? You're crowned, so you can scurry all over the board, but all you do is run. Back up, run away, back up, run away, until finally you are cornered and surrender the game. Now think about how you fight anxiety. . . .

When your strategy is to back away from events and to try to avoid certain feelings, you are using a one hundred percent defensive strategy, one that focuses completely on how to protect yourself. No one can win by only acting defensively, because you are constantly giving up ground. You have to push forward. But where are you going?

Always Fight For, Not Against

Taking control of panic is a positive process. We all have images of how we would like our lives to turn out. We consider tasks we wish to accomplish, pleasures we hope to enjoy, relationships we want to prosper. By gaining control over panic you get to turn your sights toward the positive future.

Panic, however, has other plans for you. It invites you to stop whatever else you are doing and fight against it. If you will reflect for a moment, I think you can appreciate just how much time and attention you devote to dreaded anticipation. Panic would like you to halt your life and think of nothing else except your struggle with it. In a paradoxical way, panic lives off your willingness to fight it or run from it.

Don't fall for this trap. Never fight against this invisible enemy. Where can you place your attention when you pull it away from your anxious anticipation? When you become anxious, tense, or panicky, apply the skills you are learning in these chapters, but always keep an eye on your positive future—whether for today, this week, this year, or your life—to continue moving forward. Then fight forward, toward your positive goals. There are so many valuable things to be doing with your attention. The world outside you offers beautiful, warm, sunny days in the summer and the soft glow of a fire in the winter, the embraces and laughter shared with those who love you, the challenges of solving problems at work and home, the stimulating interest of conversation, music, study. Turn your attention outside yourself. Become connected to life and allow that rich healing contact to influence your feelings. Stop trying to figure yourself out! Be anxious and simultaneously become interested in your surroundings.

Let me illustrate this point with an analogy. Let's say that you have had a busy, active week. It's now Friday afternoon. Tomorrow, company will arrive for a weekend visit. You would like to prepare by cleaning the house and doing some laundry but at the same time you feel physically fatigued from the week.

What do you do? One choice is to focus on your fatigue. "I'm not going to let this exhaustion beat me. I'm going to fight that couch, because I want so much just to lie down and sleep." Notice the way your attention turns to the negative: how to stop exhaustion from setting in, how to keep yourself from taking a rest. You waste energy in this struggle.

Another choice is to look toward the positive future. "I would like my home to appear clean tomorrow. I also want to feel rested. Most important, I want to enjoy my guests over the next two days." When you look forward to your desired goals, your attitude shifts. Perhaps in the long run it is best that you take that nap right now so that you will feel more like cleaning in a couple of hours. Or maybe doing a quick pickup and hiding that dirty laundry in a closet will give you more time to relax and enjoy your friends. Fighting exhaustion is no longer the issue. Straightening up a bit, feeling rested, and having a pleasurable weekend are much more important.

In that same way, when anxiety or panic arrives, keep your attention on your positive goal while you respond. In essence, your attitude is, "I am going to continue in this direction. Right now I need to see how I can support myself while I'm feeling uncomfortable. I'll take as long as I need to support myself so that I can continue heading toward my goal."

Taking Back Territory

You and I are working on a very specific protocol to support you when you are uncomfortable. It is an aggressive approach to taking control of your anxiety attacks. Think of this as a strategy to take back the territory that rightly belongs to you: where you travel, how long you stay, who you share time with, what job you accept, what emotions you feel, what goals and dreams you reach for. We will do this by advancing into threatening territory and making it safe for you again.

The general rule is this: The more aggressively you can face your distress and doubt, the more powerfully you will win back your life. We've been addressing two major changes to your reaction to help you toward this goal. You adopt a stance of "I want to face uncertainty and discomfort." You also take on an attitude of "I can handle whatever happens." You then match your actions with these attitudes: you go toward what you have been avoiding. This approach is counterintuitive. You have to embrace the role of risk-taker, because you head straight at your fear of discomfort and doubt.

If trying to get rid of anxiety and panic tends to keep them around, then what would happen if you did the opposite, if you encouraged them to stay? (I can hear you now: "What!? I'm not even going to *listen* to this one!") Keep in mind that this is a mental game. Panic gains territory as long as it gets you to react in a specific way. If you change your reaction, then you start taking territory back.

Stronger and Longer

You now know what happens when you face your doubt and distress by saying and believing, "I want this." We are going to escalate that position to:

- I want it to be strong.
- I want it to last.

Remember the research on habituation: You overcome a fear by frequently facing it, with strong enough distress, for long enough. Those three characteristics allow the body-&-mind to develop a habit of exposure to threat that will diminish your fear. You and I, however, have a secret tactic that few people use. It is a powerful strategy that will speed up your progress: the mindset of *wanting* whatever experience you face.

Here is one way to think about the logic behind wanting to be strongly uncomfortable and uncertain for an extended time:

- Since you *need* to frequently face your fears and your distress for an extended period to get better, and . . .
- You *want* to get better, then . . .

- You should *want* frequent, intense, long exposure to your fears, even though it is uncomfortable.

People tend to give themselves a mixed message before they practice facing their fears: "I don't want to go in there and get anxious, but I know I have to to get better. So I will." Notice how this directly expresses their resistance. Resistance is the biggest roadblock to your progress. If you take this mindset, you are complying with an expectation ("I should do this"), but your heart isn't in it. You are subordinating yourself to the role of passive, disconnected follower of some instruction manual.

As I encourage you to face your fears, pick up this frame of mind instead:

I am so committed to getting better that I'm willing to go out there and get anxious. If I don't get anxious, I'm not practicing. If I don't practice, I won't get better. I really want to get better, so I actually *do* want to get anxious (even though it scares me) in order to practice my skills. I want my anxiety to stick around (even though I don't like it at all), because I want to learn to tolerate my anxiety in this situation. And (gulp!) for this practice to count toward my progress, it is important for me to want my anxiety to be strong. I want this practice to count, so I want my anxiety to get strong here. (But it's not going to be pleasant!)

Now, of course, you don't have to be that wordy every time you practice. I'm just trying to create the point of view to direct your actions. You can truncate all that talk down to this simple message:

I want my discomfort and doubt to show up, to be strong here, and to last for a while. I *want* to do that hard work because I want to get better.

What's the Secret?

I said this attitude is a secret tactic; now let me tell you the secret. By honestly wanting strong physical sensations or strong doubt, by wanting them to last, by wanting to have them frequently, you will improve more rapidly. Why? Because you are not resisting. When you give up resisting, magic happens. Over time, you will notice that you spontaneously start feeling more in control. Once again, though, the magic comes paradoxically: If you are looking for feeling in control, you won't find it. Your job is simply to do your work: to practice wanting frequent episodes of strong sensations or doubt that last a while.

So look for discomfort, look for a feeling of doubt, hope that they will stick around and feel strong, and be surprised when you eventually get positive results. Start seeking out opportunities to get uncomfortable. That's how you should think about threatening events—as opportunities. Look for them every day, in everything you do: "Is there a chance I can practice feeling uncomfortable here? I hope so."

In any situation, if you notice yourself suddenly feel threatened and scared, that's your cue to tell yourself, "This looks like a good opportunity to practice." When you declare these moments as your time to practice, then you are in control, not panic. Plus, you have a definition of practice that directs your actions and reactions: You are looking for discomfort to stay strong and to linger.

When you notice yourself spontaneously feeling uncomfortable, talk to yourself about how to respond. You might say something like this: "Boy, I don't feel good. I'm scared about how long this might last. I'm scared about this getting stronger. OK . . . so . . . time to practice. If I'm going to practice now, then I'm going to practice with the attitude of wanting these feelings to stick around and be pretty strong."

Look for opportunities to practice daily. You might structure your practices similar to these two examples.

. . .

If you know you're in good heart health but still worry about your heart beating too fast, possibly leading to a heart attack, then go to the gym and start peddling on a stationary bike. When your heart accelerates, you'll probably feel scared. Tell yourself something like, "Whew! I'm worried about my heart now. But that's what I'm doing here, trying to get uncomfortable. Good. Now I want to stay scared. I'll set a goal to pedal for 30 minutes while I'm afraid. Tough as that sounds, I'm going to shoot for it." After 5 minutes you might hear yourself say, "Oh, no, how do I know whether I'm going to have a heart attack? This could be too much for me!" What do you say then? "OK, there's my doubt. I'm looking for this sense of threat. I want these thoughts to pop up. This is going in the right direction. (And I'm scared!)"

. . .

You decide to tackle your fear of driving on the interstate. You plan a practice: You will get onto the highway, drive 3 miles to the next exit (something you haven't done in 12 months), get off, drive across the bridge and get back on, heading toward your original exit. As you anticipate the practice, you have doubts that you can do it. "Good. There's my doubt; I'm wanting that." Then just sit with your uncertainty for a bit. Don't embellish your negative thoughts or talk yourself out of them. Just let go of your attachment to them and know they'll be back momentarily. When you're ready, head out on the drive. When your anxiety gets stronger: "Yikes! Oh, yeah, I want this. I can handle this. I'd like this feeling to stick around." If your distress feels overwhelming and you can't get perspective on that fear, then perhaps you can pull over onto the side of the highway and take a break. Tell yourself, "It's great I just practiced such a challenge. It's only practice; it's not a test, no matter how I do. I'll sit here and recover for a bit and then finish the practice." To the best of your ability, drive that same six-mile circuit between those same two exits three or four times in a row. You can take a break between each lap if you want. Then you will have a 30- to 60-minute practice under your belt. That counts! Do that practice several times in one week and you have the therapeutic package: experiencing and wanting frequency, intensity, and duration of distress and doubt.

Practice Wanting Intense, Long Threatening Events

As you begin to seek out these threatening events, here is a critical instruction: You do not need to do anything to cause your distress to become stronger or last longer except to go toward the events that have threatened you in the past. Don't try to feel more anxious. Don't try to become more confused or uncertain. Only focus on wanting your discomfort and doubt, without trying to make them happen. Allow them. Invite them. If they show up, great! If they don't show up, great! You will still be practicing, regardless of your anxiety level.

What else should you do? Simply enter the situation and attempt to act as close as you can to the way a person would normally act in such a context. When driving, pay attention to your basic driving skills. If you're shopping, focus on finding and purchasing your desired items. At lunch with a friend, attend to ordering your food, engaging in conversation, and enjoying your meal to the best of your ability. When you become aware of your anxiety, welcome it. Subvocalize that message by saying something like, "Good, I want to be anxious here." Then return your attention to the task of driving or shopping or having lunch with your friend. If you notice an increase in your anxiety, respond to your awareness with a message such as, "I just got more anxious.

Whew—scary! But good, because I was looking for more distress." Focus back on your task. If your anxiety stays around: "Good, I want my anxiety to last as long as possible." Then turn your concentration, as best you can, back to your task.

Again, let me repeat: As long as you are stepping into the scenes that threaten you, you don't need to increase the intensity of sensations or worry. Nor do you need to cause your distress and doubt to continue. Your job is to *want* those changes. We are working on shifting your attitude toward sensations and thoughts when you anticipate them or when you start experiencing them. Create within you a welcoming state of mind. When you mistakenly hope that your distress and doubt won't increase or linger, you will be throwing fuel on the fire. To paradoxically seek out and want those experiences is a way of robbing that fire of oxygen. Go toward doubt and distress and you will master them.

To win over anxiety, you stop fighting it. To rid yourself of panic, you let it exist. To gain control of doubt, you stop resisting it. And that is the paradox.

PRACTICE YOUR SKILLS

Wanting Intense, Long Threatening Events

1. Look for a situation where you can provoke anxiety and doubt.
2. Remind yourself that you can cope with any consequences. If you are unsure how you will cope, then work that out before you begin. Remember, your best stance is this one: "Whatever happens here, I'll handle it." Work on getting to that attitude before you enter the situation.
3. As you anticipate the event and as you are entering the event, remind yourself of your goals:

   • "I want to feel uncomfortable here."
   • "I want to feel uncertain how this will unfold."

- "I'm looking for my distress and doubt to be strong."
- "I'd like my anxiety and uncertainty to last as long as possible."

4. Focus your attention on your chosen task, whether it is driving, shopping, watching a movie, or talking to someone.

5. Anytime you notice and feel threatened by anxiety and doubt, remind yourself: "I want this. I'd like it to stick around." Then return your attention, to the best of your ability, back to your chosen task.

6. Expect that you will repeatedly become distracted by your fearful thoughts, to the degree that you may have difficulty concentrating or performing your chosen task. Do the best you can to forge ahead anyway. Be willing to sacrifice concentration and competence.

7. If you must end your chosen task because of your distress or fear, then support your efforts and your courage for the practice you completed.

When to Move to the Next Skills

Practice applying these principles as often as possible. Several times daily would be great. Set as your goal to practice these attitude skills until you can consistently apply them to your threatening situations. Before you move on to the next skills, accomplish the tasks listed below.

How Do You Know You Are Succeeding?

☐ You are actively looking for frequent opportunities to practice provoking anxiety and doubt.

☐ You are willing to cope with any of your feared consequences of the event.

☐ You commit to your practice goals of
 ☐ wanting to be uncomfortable and uncertain
 ☐ wanting your discomfort and doubt to be strong
 ☐ wanting your discomfort and doubt to last for an extended period of time
☐ You expect that your distress and doubt might cause you to perform your chosen task at a suboptimum level. You accept that.
☐ When you become uncomfortable or uncertain, you can remind yourself those are the feelings you are seeking. You allow them but don't react by fighting them or trying to get rid of them.
☐ When you end your practice, regardless of what you accomplished, you support your courage and effort.

As you practice, don't be disappointed by early struggles to apply these concepts. They are new, and they are a challenge to your instinctual response; therefore, they are supposed to be difficult to apply. But once this special attitude is in place, your entire perspective will shift. Accepting and inviting anxiety is the goal here, rather than being free of anxiety. Panic comes when we try to control our anxiety and we fail. Since you are no longer fighting with your uncomfortable sensations, it is much harder to experience a sense of failure. When you stop saying, "I am failing right now," panic won't be able to dominate you.

CHAPTER 13

Stand without Crutches

Can you relate to these scenarios?

. . .

You make a commitment for lunch with a friend, but later you begin to feel uneasy about it, so you ask your spouse to come along for support. Now, as you nervously wait in the restaurant lobby, you place two fingers on your wrist and after a few seconds start shaking your head. "My pulse is racing. I don't know about this. . . ." You check in your pocket for the anti-anxiety pill, just in case. The lunch goes better than you expected, and you leave feeling relieved.

. . .

You venture out onto the highway, even though driving in traffic has caused you problems in the past. You can hear your mind working up a good case for panic. "I can't do this. This is really frightening. I could lose control." But you don't want to quit, so you engage your usual distractions. As you turn on the radio, you begin a drone of diversion, "I can do this. I can do this. I can do this." And every few minutes you intersperse that reassurance with a breathing skill. "If I can just keep taking a good Calming Breath, I'll be fine." You make it to your destination and back again, feeling thankful that you survived this near miss with panic.

Your Safety Crutches

In both examples, the individuals have generated a set of coping strategies to allow them to tolerate events that they would otherwise avoid. That's commendable. I call these safety crutches because you lean on them for your sense of security. The biggest crutch people use is to avoid threatening situations altogether. The second is to escape as they sense they are about to panic. But there are dozens of subtle ways that people avoid uncertainty and discomfort. I've listed many of the common safety crutches at the end of this chapter. Here are the ones from the previous scenarios:

- Asking a supportive person to accompany you
- Checking your pulse
- Carrying an anti-anxiety pill
- Distracting yourself
- Repeating reassuring phrases
- Engaging in relaxation exercises

Crutches are essential when you are first healing a broken leg. But if you want to walk independently again, you eventually have to put those crutches away. And so it is with panic: When you are choosing to take a giant step into a new, threatening arena, crutches can be quite handy. If you haven't taken a commercial flight in six years because of severe panic attacks, and next week you have to fly across country, then traveling with a friend, taking anti-anxiety medications, practicing calming skills, and bringing music, magazines, and Sudoku puzzles to refocus your attention—these sound like good ideas to me. But if you continue to use crutches on all your flights from now on, "just in case," then you can never overcome your fear of panic.

Why Bother?

Why should you reduce your reliance on safety crutches? There are two ways that crutches interfere: they weaken your sense of control and they decrease your ability to gain control in threatening situations. To feel free of panic's threats, you will need to challenge the presumed benefits of those crutches. Let me summarize what we are learning from research studies. Open your mind to the possibility of these two points, since they seem opposite of logic.

1. *Using safety crutches makes you feel more vulnerable to anxiety. Facing threat directly makes you feel stronger.*

Your solution—to use safety crutches—perpetuates your problem. Anything that you do with the conscious intent to avoid threat will reconnect you with that threat. While you are consciously thinking, "I'm so glad the traffic is light," you will unconsciously think, "because if it were heavy right now, I'd be terrified!" The natural response to threat is anxiety, so even though you are reassuring yourself, you are simultaneously scaring yourself into believing that driving in traffic is dangerous.

Three studies have been conducted with healthy individuals who have no anxiety-related disorders. The subjects in the experiments were asked to generate uncomfortable physical sensations—for instance, by breathing in oxygen with a mix of carbon dioxide or by hyperventilating. In all three studies, those who were prone to use crutches to distract themselves from their discomfort reported more panic symptoms and felt less in control than those who paid attention to their sensations.

It's not that people using safety crutches are actually more anxious. Their heart rate fluctuations during practice tend to be the same as those who face anxiety directly. But they rate their sensations to be stronger. That means using crutches may cause you to perceive that you are more uncomfortable than you actually are. Who needs that?!

2. *When you pay attention to your discomfort and doubt, you improve.*

Researchers have extensively studied the benefits of staying aware of your discomfort and your fears when you face a threatening situation. Yes, trying to get your mind off your discomfort can give you some relief for the moments while you are practicing, but in the long run it keeps you stuck. In one study, six months after completing treatment, the group that was willing to focus on their discomfort continued to report greater improvements than the group distracting themselves with safety crutches.

In one study, people with claustrophobia (fear of closed-in spaces) were instructed to face their threatening situations during treatment. One group was asked to focus on their perceived threats during their practice. A second group was given a complicated mental task to keep their minds busy and away from thinking about their fears. In other words, they were trained to use a safety crutch. The group directly facing their threat were able to reduce their fear significantly more than the group engaged in distraction.

In another study, people with claustrophobia were asked to enter into a closed-in place alone to practice tolerating the feared situation. One group was instructed that they could use safety crutches any time they needed them during the practice. They were permitted to open a window if they desired fresh air, to stand by the door so they could get out quickly, to check that the door was unlocked whenever they wanted, and they could speak with the experimenter through an intercom. The other group was offered no safety crutches. The experimenter instructed them on the benefits of focusing on their perceived fears to discover whether they were true threats. It was much easier for this second group to overcome their claustrophobic fears. Using the safety crutches ended up working against the progress of the first group.

What does that mean? *You get better when you are willing to be anxious and uncertain.* You have to face short-term discomfort and doubt for long-term improvement. You need to *not know* how strong your anxiety will become and go forward anyway. You need to *not be sure* whether there will be negative consequences. This is because you must *challenge your belief* that something intolerable is going to occur. How? By putting yourself in that circumstance and discovering what happens.

Think carefully about what I am saying. The research shows that there is an excellent way for you to improve. Dozens of studies have led us to this conclusion: Permitting yourself—even encouraging yourself—to be scared, and feeling that fear instead of blocking it, is healing. These findings have held up in studies of people with panic disorder, post–traumatic stress disorder (PTSD), obsessive-compulsive disorder, claustrophobia, social anxiety, and phobias of driving, heights, and small animals. It is clear that distracting yourself is not in your best interest.

For example, one study involved thirty-seven women who had been assaulted. All of them developed PTSD, and the study looked at how well they improved after treatment. The treatment protocol, called exposure, involved repeatedly imagining the assault while a trained therapist supported their efforts. While this is an excellent, well-researched form of therapy for PTSD and all the women improved, there was a significant finding. The women who allowed themselves to feel very scared while they were practicing the exposure and who didn't block those feelings when they noticed them, were eight times more likely to improve to the highest stage of functioning afterward. *Eight times more likely* to get better—that is a highly significant finding.

So test out your theory that something bad is going to happen, and test it out without any crutches. If you can have faith that such a protocol will help in the long run, you will be more willing to tolerate your anxiety and doubt in the short run.

Get Rid of the Option

Having *access* to safety crutches, even if you don't use them, limits your progress just as much as if you use them. Perceiving that you have the option to lean on a crutch during practice interferes with your ability to learn to handle anxiety to the same degree as actually leaning on it. Carrying that anti-anxiety pill in your pocket "just in case" seems like more progress than taking the pill, and that's true. But to finish your work, you may need to practice without the option of that pill to bail you out of trouble. Carrying a cell phone or a list of coping skills, preparing excuses for leaving, knowing how to reach a support person, constantly reassuring yourself—these are all just-in-case crutches that cause you to avoid facing your fears directly. They perpetuate your belief that the threat is real and valid.

Breaking the Cycle

Here is the pattern you use to strengthen your fear, which I've illustrated in Figure 4. When you face an event that you perceive as threatening (1), you grab one or more of your crutches (2) and feel some immediate relief (3). But as you mentally register that relief, you simultaneously (even if you don't notice this) conclude that you averted an experience that could have been dangerous (4) if you hadn't used your crutch (5). This causes you, at least unconsciously, to again associate the event with danger (6). Now your fear about the event becomes stronger (7) in an ever-reinforcing cycle.

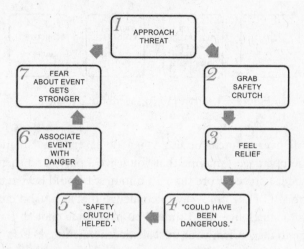

Figure 4. Safety crutches in the cycle of fear.

For instance, as you approach that lunch date with your friend and perceive it as a threat, you ask your spouse to come along, you monitor your heart rate, and check for your medication. These crutches offer you some incremental degree of relief, but, perhaps outside of your awareness, you have a sense of how bad that scene might have been. You continue through the event. When it's over, you continue to feel reassured that those crutches "worked" because you averted disaster. The next time you approach a similar scene, your fear-of-threat returns, and you begin reaching for your crutches again.

Here's how to pay attention to your anxiety and your perceived threat. I've illustrated it in Figure 5 on the next page.

Consider approaching that same threatening event (1). When you have the urge to use a safety crutch, hold back (2). Instead, tolerate your anxiety sensations and be willing to directly face your doubt about what bad might happen. Believe that you will figure out how to cope with whatever comes your way, as we worked on in the earlier chapters (3). Then let yourself discover what actually happens in the scene (4).

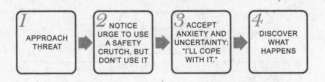

Figure 5. Learning to cope without crutches.

With every crutch you use, you add a layer of invalidation of your competence. Imagine that you leave a party and then say, "Maybe if I stayed more than 30 minutes, I would have humiliated myself." The only way to challenge that as a valid conclusion is to stay longer next time. You have to *do* enough for *long* enough to disconfirm your unrealistic, threatening beliefs.

Your goal is to challenge any unrealistic beliefs that you have about how such events will unfold. You don't know if those unrealistic beliefs are true or false, and that thought will make you anxious. Good. That's what we're looking for: Go forward into a threatening situation, while feeling uncomfortable and uncertain, and discover what happens in the scene. You must face the situation without those crutches to discover that you can cope. With time and practice, you will have fewer and fewer doubts about your ability to cope.

As you practice, remember that you aren't just focusing on your fear of how anxious you might get. The bigger threat is what you imagine will happen next. You will grab on more tightly to any safety crutch that you think will prevent your feared catastrophes—running out of the grocery store, fainting, causing a scene, having a heart attack. You must practice to test out those theories, not just practice to find out if your uncomfortable sensations fade away.

How do you do that? When you decide to practice, to the best of your ability, don't do anything to save yourself from embarrassment, or to reduce your anxiety, or to feel more secure. Do nothing to hide your anxiety or to improve your performance. If sweat is getting in your eyes as you give that speech, take a moment to wipe your brow, then keep going. If you get lost or confused, pause to look back at your notes, then push on. Just be yourself in the moment, and focus on the task at hand, whether it is making the point to your audience or wiping the sweat from your face. Then discover what happens and how you cope with it. Whatever you learn, apply that to your next encounter with threat.

In Form 1 of Chapter 11 (page 207) you generated a list of opportunities to practice your skills. Use Form 3 below to create a list of safety crutches you use for each event. When you are ready to experiment with your coping abilities, this will give you a sense of your typical crutches. Work over time to eliminate as many of those crutches as you can.

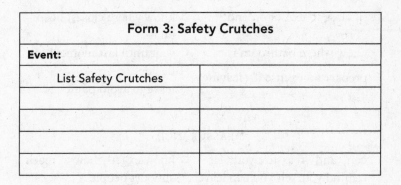

Form 3: Safety Crutches	
Event:	
List Safety Crutches	

SAFETY CRUTCHES

SECURITY PROPS

- ☐ carry cell phone
- ☐ carry anti-anxiety pill
- ☐ carry water
- ☐ bring friend or family member
- ☐ carry phone numbers to call in "emergency"
- ☐ carry book or other distraction object

RELAXATION

- ☐ try to stay relaxed
- ☐ depend on relaxation skills
- ☐ depend on breathing skills

MONITORING

- ☐ monitor thoughts
- ☐ check pulse
- ☐ check breathing
- ☐ try to swallow
- ☐ time symptoms
- ☐ watch clock
- ☐ check weather

ESCAPE & ESCAPE PLANS

- ☐ sit close to exit or on end of row
- ☐ know where bathroom is
- ☐ prepare an excuse for leaving
- ☐ know where closest hospital is
- ☐ wait until last moment to decide
- ☐ leave to avoid panic

REASSURANCE

- ☐ constantly reassure yourself
- ☐ remind yourself you can leave
- ☐ get reassurance from others
- ☐ repeatedly rehearse a behavior
- ☐ know exactly how to reach support people
- ☐ practice only with someone familiar
- ☐ frequently visit doctors

STABILITY

- ☐ hold on to cart or someone's hand
- ☐ lean against wall
- ☐ sit instead of stand
- ☐ stand or walk within reach of wall or other support
- ☐ tense up to keep control

LIMIT OR RESTRICT PRACTICE

- ☐ do something hurriedly
- ☐ do something briefly
- ☐ practice only when confident you won't be anxious
- ☐ do activities only at certain times/certain days (i.e., avoid rush hour)
- ☐ practice only when feeling well-rested and calm
- ☐ hope that symptoms won't last much longer
- ☐ make "5 more minutes" bargains

DISTRACT YOURSELF

- ☐ keep radio turned up
- ☐ talk constantly
- ☐ make support person talk constantly
- ☐ listen to music or read a book
- ☐ close eyes
- ☐ look at floor
- ☐ sing songs to yourself
- ☐ repeat "it's only anxiety"

LIMIT OR BLOCK SYMPTOMS

- ☐ seek fresh air
- ☐ roll down the window in the car
- ☐ don't eat
- ☐ don't exercise "too much"
- ☐ stay in right hand lane
- ☐ never pass a car
- ☐ carry list of coping skills
- ☐ keep reading list of coping skills
- ☐ block worried thoughts
- ☐ take anti-anxiety pill "just in case"
- ☐ drink alcohol
- ☐ sip water

PROTECT FROM OTHERS

- ☐ don't make eye contact
- ☐ don't talk to people
- ☐ practice with few people around
- ☐ avoid crowds

CHAPTER 14

Talk to Panic

I can still remember Mary B.'s words: "Come on, panic, give me your best shot." Here's how she set the scene. "I was at the library gathering some research for a paper. After about twenty or thirty minutes I suddenly started feeling quite anxious and confined. I really wanted to run out of there. My body started shaking, I felt light-headed and I lost all concentration on my work. Then, I don't know how it came to me, but I decided to take the bull by the horns. I walked to the end of the row of shelves and sat down cross-legged on the floor. (I didn't want to crack my head open if I fainted.) Then I said, 'Come on, panic, give me your best shot.' And I just sat there. I sat there and took it. Within two or three minutes all the symptoms stopped. I got up and finished my work, which required about three more hours in the library."

That was quite a learning experience for Mary B. Before that night she would have left the building immediately upon noticing her uncomfortable sensations, gone straight home, never finished that research, and mentally kicked herself over the next two or three weeks for having failed at her task. Instead, through her courageous effort (remember, she feared that she might faint and injure herself), she learned a powerful lesson: If you transform your reaction to your experience, you transform your experience.

Changing the Rules

Now I'm going to teach you the skill that Mary B. used. Consider this an advanced skill, because it involves a leap of faith to create this transformation. Not everyone will be willing to try this out, and it isn't a required skill. But I can tell you this: when it works, people report that it works in a powerful way. If you are up for the challenge, let's get started.

Certainly panic and anxiety are not the enemy. They are your body-&-mind's response to what you perceive as threatening situations. However, to learn this next skill, consider anxiety and panic as entities outside of you. Think of them as "panic showing up," "anxiety intruding in my concentration," "panic saying 'don't leave the house,'" or "anxiety telling me that I can't handle this." Consider panic and anxiety as challengers to your competence and autonomy, as though their job is to intimidate you into staying stuck and avoidant. If you venture out, if you take risks, they want to scare you back to your place of safety. They want you to believe that as long as you play by their rules, they will back away and leave you alone. Only you know the rules they have provided you, but they are probably similar to these:

- Control your breathing; don't get out of breath.
- Stay calm; don't get dizzy, weak, or nauseous or have a rapid heart rate.
- Don't feel trapped; always be able to escape quickly.
- Don't lose control or get confused or cause a scene.
- Know exactly how things will turn out, or don't do them.
- Don't embarrass yourself or others.
- Don't let people see you having difficulty.
- Don't venture out of your safe area.

- Don't go without your safety crutches (your partner, your cell phone, a ready excuse to leave, etc.)

Panic and anxiety direct your actions through voice commands. You could even say they commandeer your voice. If you listen in, you will hear yourself subvocalize the messages,

"I better not ____."

"I can't handle ____."

"I hope no one notices ____."

"I'll be trapped if I ____, and I can't let myself be trapped."

And there you have it! As long as you listen to these voice commands and follow their rules—by avoiding—panic and anxiety will leave you alone. But what have you sacrificed? You know already: your freedom, your pride, your sense of accomplishment, and so many pleasures in life.

It's time to stop playing by panic's rules. We've already been working on this strategy by going toward what you fear and wanting to experience what you have been guarding against in the past. In Chapter 12, I introduced you to "I want it to be strong, and I want it to last." Now we're going to add an interesting little mind game into the mix. We are going to fool around with specifically how you are talking in your mind and who you are talking to. Instead of talking to yourself, you are going to subvocalize instructions to panic. Here is the process:

1. When you get distracted, preoccupied, or threatened by your fearful thoughts, literally speak to panic or anxiety as though it exists outside your sense of yourself.

2. Give it instructions about what to do. Make sure the instruction is opposite of what it expects.

3. Then return to your current activity. Don't listen for a response to your instruction. Don't wait for a reaction.

Don't look for any benefit from what you just said. Disengage your attention from your sensations or worry, and attend to your desired actions. Make your request of panic, then immediately turn back to your task.

4. When anxiety grabs your attention again (which might occur within seconds), be OK with that and return to Step 1.

In the following chart you'll see some examples. In the first column are experiences you might worry about. In the second column are typical fearful responses to each sensation in the first column. For it to survive, panic needs you to respond to sensations by becoming threatened and hoping it won't hurt you further. In the past, you did whatever it asked as long as it quieted your anxiety. That last column holds examples of how to change your commenting, taking a position opposite of what panic needs to hear. Notice that I label the last column "How to instruct panic." Your job now is to turn the tables on your anxiety, to change the rules, to take a stance that will be totally unfamiliar to panic. Make a request of panic that is absolutely opposite of what it requires to survive. Instead of looking for ways to placate it, you should give it an assignment, as though you are in charge. Tell it what to do, from a one-up position, not a one-down. "Give me more. That's not strong enough. Make it stronger." Instead of going along with panic's game plan, challenge the plan, and provoke a reaction. What reaction do you get? As Mary B. illustrated, very often panic becomes "confused" and doesn't know how to react. Thus the struggle begins to take new shape.

There you go again with your reaction to my ideas: "What!? Are you nuts!? I suffer from a serious problem of debilitating anxiety attacks. These suggestions are demeaning. And crazy! And they can't possibly help." But hold on there, give me a chance. Paradoxical interventions do sound crazy. You're going to need to operate on faith here until your practice gives you some evidence that this can work.

Talking to Panic

Sensation	What panic needs to hear	How to instruct panic
Increased heart rate	"If my heart speeds up, I won't be able to stand it."	"Please, panic, make my heart beat faster. Now!"
Lightheaded-ness	"Oh, no. I'm going to faint."	"I am nowhere near light-headed enough. More, please."
Confusion	"I can't ask that question. They'll know how confused I am."	"Can you make me so confused that I can't put a sentence together? And could you hurry up, please?"
Weak legs	"I've got to lean on something before I fall."	"Jelly legs. I want jelly legs. Please make my legs collapse underneath me! If you could throw in slamming my head on the floor, I'd appreciate it."
Panic	"I could have a heart attack!"	"Come on, panic, is that all you got? Give me your best shot!"
Hands shaking	"If they notice, I'll be humiliated."	"Panic, I beg you, make my hands shake so much that people can see them shaking from the back of the auditorium."

Reflect back on what Mary B. did. She had already learned the following: It's OK to experience anxiety; I can even handle a panic attack; I want to approach these problem situations instead of avoiding them. And she had already practiced those attitudes out in her world; that's how she knew they helped her. Given those lessons, it wasn't a big step over to her request for panic to "give me your best shot." What happened when she took that active stance? The sensations subsided within a few minutes, and she continued with her valued task.

I know that some of you are choosing to read through this entire set of chapters before you do any practice. That's fine. However, since you have not yet mastered the earlier skills, it

RESISTING (this is where you started) ⇩	"This is bad and wrong." "I don't want this!" "I can't handle this!"
WANTING DISCOMFORT & UNCERTAINTY (Chapter 11) ⇩	"It's OK that I'm anxious right now." "I want this." "I can handle this."
WANTING <u>MORE</u> DISCOMFORT & UNCERTAINTY (Chápter 12) ⇩	"I want it to be strong." "I want it to last."
TALKING TO PANIC (where we are now)	"Come on, panic, give me your best shot!" "Can't you, please, give me more doubt?" "Make this sensation stronger, now, please." "Please make this doubt continue."

may put you at a disadvantage as I introduce this skill. Experience is the greatest teacher, so you may need to work on the skills of the previous chapters before you can buy into this strategy.

But if you have been practicing along the way, and you have passed those checklists at the end of Chapters 11 and 12 called "How do you know if you are succeeding?" then this step can feel like a natural progression. Here is where we have come from and where we are now (see table on p. 245).

Entering from the Side Door

When you are caught up in the drama of panic, you say to your body-&-mind, in essence, "This is going to be awful! Protect me." Of course, being a well-trained fighting machine, your body-&-mind responds by going into fight-flight-or-freeze mode. In this new strategy, while you are busy engaging panic in a reversal of roles, you are simultaneously communicating to your body-&-mind. You are overriding that emergency message, telling your body-&-mind, "It's OK; I've got a handle on this. I'm going to play a game here. Alarm mode isn't necessary. You can relax your guard." Your task is to convey to your autonomic nervous system—with its fight-flight-or-freeze response—that it can stand down, it does not need to secrete any more epinephrine to protect you. You are not at risk and don't need your nervous system to remain on guard.

However, giving your body-&-mind that message directly (talking to yourself) is not always the most effective way to accomplish the task of managing your anxiety. To unlearn this pattern of scaring-yourself-&-then-going-on-guard takes finesse. That's why, with the experience you now have of wanting what you have been afraid to experience, I'm encouraging you to personify panic and talk directly to it. Talk the talk of someone who seeks out and wants whatever feels threatening. Racing heart? "Yes!" Dizziness? "Oh, yes, please." Confusion? "I so want that." To the best of your ability, take an extreme position:

No matter how strong the sensations, they are not strong enough and you want more. No matter how long it is lasting, how intense it is getting or how frequent it is occurring, it's not enough!

Remember that your goal is to override an alarm system that is instinctual. It is a powerful, primitive, and automatic defense system. It is responding impeccably, but it is responding to a false message of "this is dangerous." When you congruently convey that you don't need rescuing, it will gladly step aside. It takes many repetitions of this message to sink in (because part of you will continue to feel scared), but the body-&-mind has no interest in continuing to respond to false signals of danger. At the same time, you choose to supersede your current belief system—a set of rules—that you have adopted to protect yourself against danger.

Of course, then, if our goal is to reverse your body-&-mind's direction, and we are to challenge a powerful, dominating belief system, then we will need all the cleverness available from your creative conscious intelligence. That's how you should think of this strategy: It is purposely manipulating your unhelpful beliefs and simultaneously permitting your brain's arousal system to quiet down.

What to Believe

Begging panic to make you more anxious is not meant to be an honest communication of your desires. It is meant as a cognitive manipulation, used as a strategy to reach your desired outcome. Here is what you need to honestly believe:

- I want to get anxious.
- I want it to last.
- I want it to be strong.

You should believe those positions based on the rationalizations I gave to you in Chapters 10, 11, and 12 and based on what you learned practicing the skills within those chapters. Now I am asking you to add another stance:

> I need to be clever if I am going to change my fear-inducing beliefs and my body-&-mind's reaction to that threat. I'm going to purposely manipulate my thoughts.

Fooling around with your mental conversation is a strategy *in service of* your honest desire to permanently change your reaction to these threats. You must approach this skill with that sense of strategy. Your efforts need to be grounded in principles that make sense to you. Otherwise, you will try this skill half-heartedly. In the face of such a rigid old belief system and powerful instinctual response, a lackadaisical effort won't cut it.

What You Are Changing

The structure of this strategy appears to be on the level of changing what you are mentally saying, but that's not it. You are changing where you place your attention. Our body-&-mind is programmed to resist discomfort and uncertainty. If you have also had terribly frightening experiences with anxiety, your belief system has lined up with that goal, too. That dynamic duo of brain and belief has created a fortress of defense that directs your moment-by-moment attention. We are going to alter the direction of your attention in a dramatic enough way that new learnings can find their way into this fortress. How? Let me review the steps of "talking to panic" again, within the context of shifting your attention.

1. *When you get anxious, literally speak to panic as though it exists outside of you.*
    You are prying your attention away from its automatic focus on your worries. Your worries feed your resistance. The less you attend to your worries, the less you will resist by giving yourself

a competing task. The less you resist, the more powerful you become. And what task are you investing in? One that is weird and different for you. One that requires concentration. The more you concentrate on mastering this task, the less you attend to your worries. Yet it simultaneously keeps your attention on your discomfort and doubt. We know from the research studies we discussed in the last chapter that by attending to your doubt and discomfort without resisting them, you contribute to your healing process.

2. *Give panic instructions that are opposite of what it expects.*

You force your attention over to the task of delivering a paradoxical message. Your logic needs to be: I want to ask for more trouble as one way to combat my powerful, automatic message of "I hope I don't have more trouble." Fighting and resisting has failed you. Resisting a threat makes the threat feel worse. The best way to stop resisting is to busy yourself with the task of inviting what you fear. You might be terribly clumsy at this task, and that won't matter a bit. You can win the booby prize as the least talented student of this skill on the entire Earth. How good you are at these instructions is irrelevant. What is relevant is where you place your attention. If you will attend to the task of developing the best skills of talking to panic, then, by default, your mind will have less attention available to float over to your worries. In game theory they use a term called zero-sum. It means you only have so much of certain resources available. For instance, let's say you have limited funding for a business project. If you spend 80 percent of your money on research and development, you only have 20 percent left to produce and market the product.

Your attention operates on a similar formula, and we can take advantage of that. When panic is winning, it is because you are "spending" vast amounts of your limited conscious attention on reacting fearfully. If you consciously and powerfully engage your mind in the project of figuring out how to ask panic to increase your sensations, then, by default, you will automatically, spontaneously withdraw mental attention from your fears. So attend to this skill, as a student trying to master it, and you will discover that it serves your goal of not attending solely on how to resist. As you stop resisting, you start the healing process.

3. *Then return your attention to your current activity. Don't look for any benefit from what you just said. Turn away from your worries and back to your task.*

You have been attending to your sensations or doubts in a negative fashion—fearing them and trying to resist them. You will not be able to immediately wrestle your attention away from them. Instead, change how you attend to them (by encouraging instead of resisting). Talk to panic. Talk to it as a customer asks for another serving, as a boss demands output from a lazy subordinate, as a blackjack player asks the dealer to "hit me again."

Then turn your attention away from the transaction, gently and immediately. You are done with your fearful thoughts. Consider the transaction as complete from your vantage point. Don't expect anything back from anxiety and don't check to see if panic is responding. Re-engage in your valued task. Turn your attention back to driving your car or talking to your friend or concentrating on your work.

When you turn your attention back to your task, your belief system and your body-&-mind will perceive it, at least in the beginning, as a risk, because you have been using your attention as a defensive system—to track your discomfort. Shifting your attention away from your worries is a form of dropping your guard. So assume you will feel anxious because of your intervention. Expect that. In the learning process we all feel insecure.

4. *When anxiety grabs your attention again (which might occur within seconds), be OK with that and return to Step 1.*

Inevitably your distress will grab your attention again, usually within moments. No matter how many times it grabs you, commit to responding to it in the same manner each time. Yes, it distracts you from your task, but that is the sacrifice you must make. If you want to get stronger, you have to practice. When you practice, you will not be able to devote all your attention to the task at hand, so others might notice you are nervous, or you might not be able to track the plot of the movie, or you may miss a turn while driving. But once you have invested the time in repeating this practice, and you have learned the skill, then you will discover the benefits of no longer fighting your fears.

The Formula

Figure 6 is a simple structure for any request you make of panic. Express a desire, conveyed in a tone that you purposely choose. It can range from a soft tone ("Would you please . . . ?") to an aggressive one ("Come on! Is this the best you can do? Give me your best shot, now!"). This desire should be your direct request for anxiety or doubt to increase strength, length, intensity, or frequency ("Give me more, please") of whatever currently

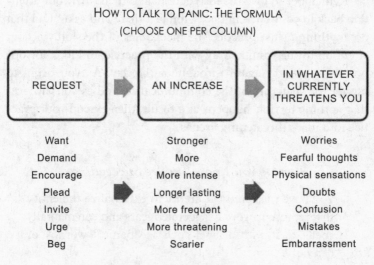

HOW TO TALK TO PANIC: THE FORMULA
(CHOOSE ONE PER COLUMN)

REQUEST	AN INCREASE	IN WHATEVER CURRENTLY THREATENS YOU
Want	Stronger	Worries
Demand	More	Fearful thoughts
Encourage	More intense	Physical sensations
Plead	Longer lasting	Doubts
Invite	More frequent	Confusion
Urge	More threatening	Mistakes
Beg	Scarier	Embarrassment

Figure 6. How to talk to panic.

threatens you, such as your bodily sensations or worries about the judgments of others.

Please note that to convey these principles as simply as possible, I have labeled them as "talking to panic." But you can give that entity any label that feels appropriate. Depending on what is threatening you, feel free to talk to "worry," "anxiety," "embarrassment," or "doubt."

Now it's time to try out this strategy. Start off with low-grade threats and low-anxiety sensations. For instance, if you have a big event tomorrow and you are beginning to notice your nervousness today, even though you are prepared, then practice talking to anxiety. Ask it (or beg it or demand it) to increase your specific uncomfortable sensations at that very moment. "(Boy, am I anxious!) Oh, anxiety, would you please make my stomach tighter? Please?" If your worries are more troubling to you: "(Geez, I'm all caught up in my worries about tomorrow.) Hey, anxiety, could you make those worries come more frequently, please? And how about making them more catastrophic? I mean, these are kind of wimpy. Really scare me, how about it!"

Remember to give the instruction, and then turn your attention back to your current task. Don't sit there and ask, "Did that do anything?" Just practice the mechanics of the skill, without attention to the results. Stay with the practice and look for opportunities to try again throughout the day. As you begin to master the structure of the communication and as you discover that nothing terrible happens as a result, then extend your practice into more threatening arenas.

How Do You Know You Are Succeeding?

☐ You have mastered the ability to externalize the entity that represents your exaggerated fears and can mentally speak to it with a label such as "panic," worry," or "anxiety."

☐ When you give instructions to panic, you understand how this is a paradoxical maneuver to train your body-&-mind to stop protecting you unnecessarily. You honestly attempt to master this strategy to move toward distress and doubt without resistance.

☐ After you make your request of panic, you are able to return to your chosen task. This does not mean that you no longer notice your discomfort; it means you can allow the sensations or thoughts to exist, without reacting to them, as you continue your valued task.

☐ You realize that distress or worries can grab your attention again within moments of when you turn away from them. You accept this and expect this. In those moments you again apply this same strategy, even if you must repeat it numerous times within a matter of minutes.

☐ You consistently practice this skill over time, without requiring that it alter what you are thinking or feeling. You know that looking for immediate changes in your experience actually contributes to your remaining stuck.

☐ If, with practice over time, you get some positive results, then you will notice that using the protocol alters your relationship with your distress and doubt. You become less intimidated by your sensations and less reactive to your worries. As awkward as this process may feel in the beginning, if you will persist through numerous repetitions, you can be successful in interrupting the drama of panic.

Support

PART IV

When You Need It

The most effective method to take control of anxiety attacks is outlined for you in Part III of this book: to be willing to face doubt and discomfort and to believe you can cope with any consequences of your actions. But you do not need to be hell-bent on racing toward all that threatens you. You can take your time, and you can build skills that will move you in the direction of confronting your fears.

These next chapters are designed for readers who feel they need more support to effectively apply the skills of Part III: Don't Panic *Live*. If you have read and tried to apply the principles of Part III and had trouble making gains, then start here. Part IV might be helpful for you if:

- You are still dominated by your negative thoughts when you get anxious and cannot get perspective.
- Your physical sensations still frighten you to the degree that you don't want to face them.

- You believe the consequences of having high anxiety or of performing below your personal standards are so great that you don't want to take that risk.
- The concepts in Part III seem too radical for your liking.

We'll work on several fronts. Once you have read through Part IV, you can focus on the specific skills that you believe will help you. The purpose of all these skills is to better prepare you to return to the strategies of Part III.

Chapter 15, "Your Mind's Observer," will explain the benefits and skills needed for mentally stepping back, away from your negative thought process. The next chapter, "Find Your Observer," will teach you about your body-&-mind's ability to slow down and to quiet down. Then, in Chapter 17, "Take a New Stance: Your Supportive Observer," you will extend the skills of the previous two chapters into a powerful internal voice that overrides your worried, hopeless, or self-critical stances and supports your courageous efforts. "Take a Hit," Chapter 18, teaches you how to tolerate your uncomfortable sensations without becoming alarmed. Chapter 19, "Face Panic," shows you how to take all your newly found skills into the world so that you can successfully face the sensations and doubts that scare you. The final chapter in this section reviews medications that may be helpful.

CHAPTER 15

Your Mind's Observer

When you face panic it's best to rid yourself of unnecessary worries or questions and replace them with a few simple thoughts.

Panic is not just uncomfortable sensations. If it caused only physical discomforts, it could disappear from your life as rapidly as it enters. Panic invades your mental processes as well. In fact, an anxious episode often begins *in reaction to* your thoughts. ("I wonder how I'll feel today? I wonder if I'll feel nervous again?") For a panic attack to grow in intensity, you must do two things:

1. You must closely observe your current experience.
2. You must comment on those observations.

Therefore, to reduce panic, consider changing either of these actions. Let's look at the two actions more closely.

Imagine that you are interested in buying a house. To begin your search, you spend a Saturday with a Realtor viewing four different houses within your size, location, and price range. At each site you will spend probably thirty to forty-five minutes walking through the rooms and around the yard. What are you doing during that time? What is your mental process?

The first thing you do is *observe*. Your eyes are scanning each room slowly: you are noticing the layout of the kitchen, the size of the bedrooms, the number of baths, and so forth. You look for moisture in the basement, insulation in the attic, and check the condition of the exterior.

Let's call this part of us that objectively gathers information our Observer. When you take a first look through a house, it is best to simply "flip on" the Observer within you. In that way you can gather much more information about each potential home. You may even take a notebook to record the facts you need to make an intelligent decision.

That's Step 1. Step 2 is to begin to comment about the data you have collected, to consider your personal preferences for size, design, and location. You analyze each house according to your needs and desires. Here is what might go through your mind as you view a house for the first time. Notice how the thoughts come in two stages:

OBSERVER: [As you drive up the driveway.] The drive is concrete; there's a two-car open garage. The house is Colonial style and the yard is manicured. COMMENT: Looks good. We could use a carport. Maybe we could enclose it one day. The outside looks well cared for. Colonials aren't my favorite, though.

OBSERVER: [As you enter the kitchen.] This is bigger than mine, with an island in the middle. Open entry into a breakfast nook. No windows in the kitchen. Also opens into the living room/dining room combo. Walk-in pantry. And lots of cabinet space. COMMENT: Wow! This is what I'm looking for! Plenty of space to spread out, plus we can eat most meals without lugging things into the dining room. And lots of storage would be a treat. Major drawback is the lack of natural light. It's so nice to be able to look outside from the kitchen. But I think I can live with it. Let's see if the rest of the house is as nice.

There is a clear and distinct difference between the Observer statements and the Comments. The Observer simply notices and reports objectively any data it receives. It is like the attitude of the judge in a courtroom: "Just the facts please, ma'am." The Observer applies no biases, preferences, personal desires, or judgments to the facts.

In Step 2 we comment on our observations. Now we are influenced by our desires, beliefs, values, hopes, fears, and judgments. ("I love it/hate it/am afraid of it/don't care for it/want it/ want to change it/doubt I can have it/wish it never happened/ hope it works," and so forth.)

Negative Observers

It is when we comment on our observations prematurely that our problems begin. Imagine that as you drove up to that house you said, "It's a Colonial. Colonials aren't my favorite. That's a strike against this house already; the inside probably won't do, either. Why don't we go on to the next one?" Your quick judgment would prevent you from continuing to gather information. In this case, you would miss the opportunity of seeing your ideal kitchen. And the quality of that kitchen might have offset the exterior design. When we are quick to judge, we lose valuable information.

Prejudice is judging people, situations, or experiences prior to objectively observing them. One of the greatest tragedies of racism, sexism, and ageism is that so many talented people are arbitrarily dismissed without regard to their unique qualities and talents. The same process occurs during panic. Our beliefs or fears are so predominant that we never objectively observe the situation. With only minimal data, we quickly interpret the situation as an emergency and begin our panic routine. We blend a two-step process into one step. We no longer take time to take advantage of our detached, objective, data-gathering Observer. Instead, we instantly analyze and interpret each new piece of information as though we were certain of its meaning.

The interpretation of events is the mental process that produces the panic response. As I discussed in Chapter 9, during a panic-provoking time the brain lacks relevant information about exactly what is going on, and it doesn't know a more appropriate way to respond. Consequently it selects the same response it used in the past to handle a similar situation. The brain pushes the panic button because we withhold new information from it. We do not slow down enough to collect current information; we fall back to our preconceived notion that we are "out of control." By using the skills of your Observer at the moment of panic, however, you can gather current, relevant information about your body and your surroundings. This vital data will guide you toward gaining control of your anxiety attack.

You already have an excellent capacity to observe. It is important to renew your acquaintance with this skill, so that you may begin to use it in a positive way during panic-provoking times.

Rather than take the time to calmly observe the threatening situation, the panic-prone person will quickly observe and interpret the situation in one swift moment. In my work with clients over the years, I have found three primary ways they "contaminate" the responsibilities of the Observer by adding negative comments during this important first step. I call the three Negative Observers the Worried Observer, the Critical Observer, and the Hopeless Observer. Let's begin with some examples of the Worried Observer's comments.

The Worried Observer

"My heart rate has increased . . . Oh no, what does that mean? Am I starting to have a heart attack? I must be."

"My speech is scheduled for next week . . . I know I'm going to start stammering. Then everyone will watch me shake in my boots. I'll be so embarrassed."

"There are a lot of people shopping here today . . . That means that the checkout lines are going to be endlessly long. I'll have to stand there forever. I'll probably start to get dizzy again. I might even faint on the spot."

The Worried Observer

- Anticipates the worst
- Fears the future
- Creates grandiose images of potential problems
- Expects and braces for catastrophe
- Watches with uneasy apprehension for any small signs of trouble

Over time, the Worried Observer creates anxiety.

The Critical Observer

"Last week when I drove to the store I had no discomfort. This morning I became anxious and never made it to the store . . . I'm doing terribly! I'm so angry I failed! I'm such a weak person."

"Tonight is the Weber's party, and I'm afraid about going . . . Well, that's typical. Every little thing bothers me! I feel like a two-year-old. When am I going to grow up and face the world!"

"They're thinking of having the family reunion in Florida . . . Oh, great. Guess who's going to spoil everything again! I'm too afraid to fly, I won't shop by myself, I don't like highways. What am I doing to this family!"

The Critical Observer

- Makes certain you understand how helpless and hopeless you are
- Doesn't hesitate to remind you of the mistakes you have made and that you are lucky to have anything or anyone in your life
- Points out each of your flaws regularly, in case you have forgotten them
- Uses any mistake to remind you of what a failure you are

Over time, the Critical Observer produces low self-esteem and low motivation.

The Hopeless Observer

"Susan wants me to go out to lunch with her . . . There's no way I can survive a restaurant. I just can't handle it. What's the point, I'll never be in control."

"I used to be so outgoing. Now I hardly leave the house unless I'm taking the kids somewhere . . . I've dug myself into a hole, and I'll be here for years."

"I feel physically drained today, and I wanted to get some work done around here . . . Why bother?"

The Hopeless Observer

- Suffers over your present experience
- Believes there is something inherently wrong with you
- Believes that you are deprived, defective or unworthy, that you are missing what it takes to succeed
- Expects that you will continue to be deprived and frustrated
- Expects that you will fail in the future just as you have failed in the past
- Believes that there are insurmountable obstacles between you and your goals

Over time, the Hopeless Observer creates depression.

All three types of negative comments contaminate your natural ability to observe. They distort information about your life in a hurtful way. They don't encourage your progress, your independence, or your self-esteem. Instead, they invite you to surrender your efforts and give in to failure.

If we study the experiences of people who have significantly restricted their lives out of fear of panic, we can hear more distinctly the destructive patterns of these Negative Observer comments. Listen to the statements of each client during one of our first sessions. Imagine how these thinking patterns literally halt their progress.

> ANN: I watch myself. I'm always trying to keep this grip on
> myself. I'm monitoring every little thing that I do, and
> in the final analysis I decide that I'm not in control.

Ann tells us that she has the skill to observe herself. But she takes that ability and moves it to a Worried Observer extreme. She becomes the detective, watching her every move to discover clues that will prove she is out of control. Since she is completely focused on herself, since she notices every small change, and since she expects the worst, sure enough, she always concludes, "I'm not in control."

> DONNA: I judge my level of success in recovery by how well
> I get through a bad feeling. If I stay out of bad feelings
> and keep going, then I feel like I'm almost healed. But if
> I lie down or quit, then I'm very negative about myself. I
> only support myself when I've been successful.

Notice that Donna, too, has that skill to observe herself. But she makes extreme interpretations of the facts. When she has a great day, she is certain her problems are over forever. Her standards are so high, however, that if she has any kind of setback she labels herself a failure. She views her actions through Critical Observer eyes, and she can never be good enough. The Critical Observer allows no room for mistakes.

> KAREN: I started to feel physically sick today, like an allergic reaction. Then I said to myself, "How much is physical and how much is psychological?" I started arguing in my mind, "Should I drive myself to therapy or not? I don't think I can." Finally I gave in to myself and asked my husband to drive me. I just didn't think I could handle it, and I didn't want to struggle anymore. Now that I'm here, a part of me doesn't really care, but another part of me feels disgusted with myself for not fighting.

Karen's statements reflect all three of the Negative Observer contaminants. Her Worried Observer questions, "Should I drive myself to therapy or not? I don't think I can." Her Hopeless Observer surrenders, "I can't handle it. I don't want to struggle anymore." Then her Critical Observer delivers the final blow, "I'm disgusted with myself for not fighting." Can you imagine what it is like to treat yourself this way on a daily basis? This is how anxiety, low self-esteem, low motivation, and depression can become the focus of a panic-prone person's life.

> SHERYLL: In my own case I'm too keen an observer, in a negative way. I'm observing myself constantly, but it's always with fear. Like Claire Weekes, a pioneer in the study of anxiety and panic says, "Headphones on your feelings."

Sheryll's Worried Observer amplifies any minor change in her feelings: "Oh, no, what was that? Is it still there? Is it getting worse? Will I be ready to handle it?" Why is she fearful? Not because she is having uncomfortable physical sensations and not because she is paying attention to her body. It is because her Worried Observer is saying to her, "Any moment now you might be overwhelmed with a severe anxiety attack. Stay on guard!" To the Worried Observer, your current experience is irrelevant. Instead, it remembers how bad the past has been and imagines how frightening the future will soon be. Your Worried Observer can actually supersede any rational thoughts. If the Worried Observer is thinking of past trauma and imagining future danger, your brain has no choice but to interpret these fantasies and not interpret your current reality. The brain then responds to the presumed danger by automatically shifting into emergency gear. *To stop the physical sensations of panic you must stop the Worried Observer from dominating your thoughts.*

> DONNA: I know I get angry with myself whenever I get tense for no reason.

There is usually some reason we get tense or anxious during a time when there is no actual threat. Either the events of the past remain with us, or we are anticipating events in the future. Using the Observer, we can objectively review those events and our reactions to them. Based on that information, we can choose the most supportive action to take. Donna's Critical Observer, however, prevents her from thinking in a caring manner about her needs. Instead it says, "There's no reason to be tense! What the hell is wrong with you!" Because her Critical Observer is so strongly embedded within her belief system, it prevents her from choosing any supportive action.

Each contaminated Observer operates on a pre-existing negative belief system. Each one of them, therefore, keeps the mind closed and prevents intelligent decision making.

> ANN: When I begin to notice symptoms I become paralyzed and I start listening in on my body. And my immediate reaction is to run away from it. I have

tried to sit or to "handle" it, but physically it depletes me so much that I have to run. I'm feeling symptoms now, and my immediate reaction is to get out of here. I don't feel I have the energy—the physical or the emotional energy—to see it through, because I've been like this for twelve years. I feel like I'm going to drop dead next week because of the effects, because of the toll this has taken on my health.

Ann's comments reflect the stance of the Hopeless Observer. She becomes "paralyzed" and completely absorbed by the uncomfortable sensations she notices. She feels so depleted of energy and imagines she will not survive. Since she has been this way for twelve years, she has decided that nothing will ever change this pattern. Every anxious episode seems to pile on top of the last one, and her burden gets heavier and heavier. Eventually, she imagines, she will collapse from the toll. This is the type of contamination that leads to depression.

Since our actions are based on our interpretation of the facts and not the facts themselves, all of the Worried, Critical, or Hopeless Observer comments prevent us from taking positive action. Turn back to the three Worried Observer examples on pages 262–263. Read each one, then imagine what action you might take in response to these interpretations. Do the same for the Critical Observer and Hopeless Observer statements. See if you notice any pattern among the nine examples. (Try it now.)

Most likely you drew some of these conclusions:

- I'd better go lie down.
- I think I'd better cancel.
- I ought to leave while I can.
- I'm not going to keep trying.
- I might as well not be around people anyway.
- I'll tell them to go without me.
- I quit.

In other words, the contaminated Observers lead to passivity and inaction. They invite you to surrender to helplessness, to stop trying, to wave the white flag.

The Worried Observer, which is usually present just before or during uncomfortable physical sensations, goes one step further. It provides a distorted interpretation of events for the brain. Take the first example: "My heart has increased its rate. Oh, no, what does that mean? Am I starting to have a heart attack? I must be." The brain makes this interpretation: "I'm losing control." The brain then responds appropriately to an inappropriate interpretation: "All systems to Emergency Response!"

That is why sometimes immediately after you ask whether uncomfortable sensations are developing, those sensations become stronger, almost magically. After such an experience you tell yourself, "Good job. I was paying close attention and caught myself before the panic snuck up on me. I'd better stay on guard more often."

But there is nothing magical about it. Do you see the vicious circle? Your "solution" creates your problem:

- You pay close attention to your physical sensations.
- You become suspicious of a minor sensation.
- You interpret that sensation to mean the beginning of an anxiety attack or other serious disturbance.
- Your brain turns on the Emergency Response to "save" you.
- You vow to be even more sensitive next time.
- You are back to Step 1.

Your Independent Observer

What is the alternative to this passive, fearful, guarded cycle? How does one get out of these old, repetitive patterns? Three general tasks are required to take control of panic-prone moments:

Step 1: Observe your experience.
Step 2: Interpret the facts.
Step 3: Choose an appropriate action.

If you can eliminate your worried, critical, and hopeless comments, your ability to observe will become one of your strongest resources.

Your Observer

- Takes time to collect all the relevant information
- Detaches from strong emotions
- May feel concern, yet thinks calmly
- Is devoid of prejudices
- Gains a perspective on the situation
- Sees problems in a different light
- Makes objective observations

Who can possibly face a challenging situation with confidence while mentally reciting a litany of fears, criticisms, or doubts? Your Observer dismisses such comments and focuses on the important information at the moment: "What is taking place in my body right now? What is special about my current situation? (Have I been afraid here before? Is it reminding me of a past or future fear?) What sense can I make of my current reaction?" You can ask and answer these questions based on a momentary reflection, as though you are briefly stepping back from the scene. ("Hmmm . . . I'm starting to get tense again. How come? Nothing special is bothering me; I'm just sitting here watching TV. [Pause for reflection.] Oh, yeah, that character on the show was just fighting with her husband. I think that's when I started getting tense.")

The ability to objectively size up a situation is a crucial first step, because this information determines what action you will take next. If, in the above example, you quickly think, "Oh, my gosh, I'm starting to have an anxiety attack. How bad will this one be?" you become a powerless victim of panic by not pausing for even a moment before surrendering to the discomfort and fear. But if instead you stop to think, "I'm reacting to the fighting on TV," now you have something you can grasp, something that seems plausible.

Gathering the facts and interpreting the facts are two different steps and should be treated as such during panic-prone times. Before you jump to any conclusions, your Observer concentrates on your present experience. It doesn't get emotional or excited. It is unattached to the facts that it gathers. Even looking around for a cause of the current tension can be done in a detached manner. Not a frantic rush of thought, such as, "Oh, I feel a little jumpy right now. I've just woken up. Why do I feel so jumpy? Oh, no, I probably didn't sleep well, or I had bad dreams. Oh, damn, here it comes, the start of another terrible day." You must remember that you have time to think methodically; "This is not an emergency." In fact, the more time you give yourself to think, the greater chance you have of using your Observer's skills.

In this example, if you are thinking with care, your Observer might say, "Hmmm . . . I'm feeling a little jumpy right now. I've just woken up. [Pause for reflection.] There is probably some logical reason I'm feeling this way, even though I'm not certain what it is." This example raises an important point. Notice that your Observer didn't come up with the exact cause of the tension. Sometimes the cause isn't obvious or immediately known. At those times your Observer makes a new factual statement: "There is some logical cause for my sensations, even though I can't put my finger on it immediately." It does not say (as the Worried Observer might), "I've got to know what's causing this, now!" Instead, it carries out its responsibility, which is to collect and report information as dispassionately as possible.

Your body may be shaking, your legs may feel weak, your breathing may be fast, but your Observer can separate itself from those sensations. It can report, in a detached manner, the facts that it gathers. It notices them but does not get preoccupied with them. *To become preoccupied with your discomfort is to encourage the discomfort.*

The Observer does not try to fix the problem. Instead, it observes the action without disturbing it. All of us who have had to react to a sudden physical emergency in the home or on the highway have first-hand experience with the skills of the Observer. After the crisis has passed, most people will be able to report in great detail everything that they saw or thought. It is as though time slowed down and every second during the crisis lasted a minute. This detailed memory is produced by our Observer. Like a video camera, it records, objectively, the relevant information. During the moment of panic, your first task will be to watch and listen through that Observer's camera.

Once your Observer has reported the facts, you can interpret them. Now you are determining the relationships among the facts you have gathered. In response to the observation about the TV show ("Oh, yeah, that character on the show was just fighting with her husband. I think that's when I started getting tense."): "Since I have trouble facing conflicts in my own life, I bet that's why I'm overreacting to this scene. I don't need to become so involved in these feelings right now."

In the second example ("Oh, I feel a little jumpy right now. I've just woken up"), one possible interpretation is, "It won't be helpful to focus on these sensations right now."

In other words, when you objectively interpret the facts you answer this question: "Based on what I now know from observing, what do I seem to need?" Again, you step back and take a calm moment to explore that thought.

In the early stages of learning this skill, I recommend that you slow down your thinking. Take at least ten times (!) longer than you do now, simply to gather your information. That sounds like forever, but "slow down" is a relative term in this situation. The panic-prone person probably takes less than a second before concluding that she is losing control. *No* objective thinking takes place. In most panic-provoking moments all you need is less than twenty seconds of observing to realistically assess the situation. Another ten seconds will often be enough time for you to interpret the information. At that point you are ready to choose an appropriate action. This suggestion of thirty seconds is only to give you a general sense of the time needed. Of course, each situation and each person require varying degrees of time. Some of my clients can accomplish these steps in less than five seconds:

OBSERVER: I'm tense.
INTERPRETATION: It's OK, I can handle that.
ACTION: Take a deep breath, sigh out loud on the exhale, loosen tense muscles.

In an example requiring a little more time, our thoughts might run like this:

OBSERVER: I'm feeling anxious right now. How come? Hmmm . . . maybe it's because Jim's going on a business trip for three days. I've been nervous during those times in the past.
INTERPRETATION: I need to find a way to reassure myself these next few days.
ACTION: Why don't I talk about my concerns to Jim before he leaves. Who knows, maybe it'll help. Plus, I'll talk with Judith. Her husband travels a lot, and she'll probably have some advice. I want to have some ideas on how to cope before Jim leaves on Wednesday.

To further illustrate these two steps, let's review the nine hypothetical situations that first appeared on pages 262–264. This time I will remove the Negative Observer comments, leaving simple Observer statements (Step 1), followed by possible interpretations (Step 2). Remember that Step 2 answers the question, "On the basis of what I now know, what do I seem to need?" Specific action to take in each scenario is not presented yet; that will be Step 3.

OBSERVER: My heart rate has increased. I'm starting to worry what that means.

INTERPRETATION: This is *not* an emergency. I can quiet my worries and calm my body.

OBSERVER: My speech is scheduled for next week. Right now I'm afraid I might perform poorly.

INTERPRETATION: It's OK to be concerned about my talk. I also probably need to gain some confidence in my ability before then.

OBSERVER: There are a lot of people shopping here today. That probably means the lines will be long. I've been uncomfortable in lines before.

INTERPRETATION: This is *not* an emergency. I need to pace myself while I'm here. I want to leave here later with at least a few groceries, and I don't need to rush myself. I'll do the best I can.

OBSERVER: Last week when I drove to the store I had no discomfort. This morning I became anxious and never made it to the store.

INTERPRETATION: When I don't meet my goals, I tend to become harsh on myself. That's not helpful. I need to support myself and set a new goal.

OBSERVER: Tonight's the Webers' party, and I'm afraid about going.

INTERPRETATION: It's OK to be afraid about the party. Social events are usually tough for me, so this is normal. I'll try to stay cooled out until we leave. And maybe I can find a few tasks to focus my attention on until then.

OBSERVER: They're thinking of having the family reunion in Florida. I've been so afraid of flying that I haven't been on a plane in six years.

INTERPRETATION: Nothing is going to be decided immediately. I have time to think about my options.

OBSERVER: Susan wants me to go out to lunch with her. I often feel trapped in a restaurant.

INTERPRETATION: I need to believe that Susan will be supportive of me if we go. And I need some control over the logistics of lunch.

OBSERVER: I used to be so outgoing. Now I hardly leave the house unless I'm taking the kids somewhere.

INTERPRETATION: This pattern is hurtful to me. I need to find some activities that will help me feel better about myself.

OBSERVER: I feel physically drained today, and I wanted to get some work done around here.

INTERPRETATION: If I do nothing all day I'll end up angry with myself. I need to start by accomplishing some very small, brief tasks. I need to take one step at a time.

In the next chapter I'll teach you a variety of ways to develop and strengthen this all-important resource of stepping back and gaining perspective during a troubling time.

CHAPTER 16

Find Your Observer

For all its apparent complexity, the human body operates with great simplicity. The autonomic nervous system controls all involuntary bodily functions. Within it, the sympathetic nervous system senses a crisis then produces the Emergency Response. As is the case in most living organisms, if the human nervous system can produce a response at one extreme, it is capable of producing a response at the opposite extreme. This is a basic tenet of physics: every action has an opposite and equal reaction.

And so it is. The sympathetic response, or Emergency Response, is balanced by the parasympathetic response, what I call the Calming Response. When a crisis has passed, the brain doesn't just stop sending those emergency communications. An entirely different set of nerves sends new signals to all the affected parts of the body. Those signals tell the heart and lungs to slow down and instruct the muscles to stop contracting. The blood pressure decreases, oxygen consumption is reduced, and blood sugar levels return to normal. These restful changes take place not accidentally, not haphazardly, but by instruction.

When I ask my clients what one change they would like to see more than anything else, their response is "To feel calmer during those panicky times, so that I can think more clearly." The fact is, you already have the capacity to turn off the emergency switch—you just don't know it. You fear you are losing control, but your body has a built-in control which is yours for the asking: You can consciously activate the parasympathetic nervous system response. One central purpose of the Calming Response is to halt and reverse the sensations of the Emergency Response. Its circuits cause every internal system to return to its normal state. Thus your parasympathetic system, with controlling fibers in all the essential parts of your body, can gradually quiet down the Emergency Response.

Dr. Herbert Benson, a pioneer in medical research into this beneficial phenomenon, was the first to label this calming process the Relaxation Response. I have chosen to relabel Dr. Benson's term for one reason: to many panic-prone people, relaxation implies "letting go" or "losing control." Because of this, they resist learning skills that promote relaxation. The word is also associated with meditative practices: not moving, emptying the mind, not thinking. The truth of the matter is that relaxation exercises and meditation do work, and you will learn them next. They are excellent tools to produce the Calming Response. But these techniques of calming the mind and body can also be modified to help you as you begin to face panic. During the actual moment of panic you need skills that clear your head of extraneous thoughts, sharpen your mind, and keep you actively alert. You need the ability immediately to confront panic and regain control of your body on short notice. You'll be learning those skills too, but they are predicated on your willingness to get quiet.

Memories and Images

Before you directly learn the techniques for producing the Calming Response, reflect for a moment on times when you have naturally felt at ease, peaceful, and calm inside. Perhaps you can remember walking into a church when it was completely empty. A church can be awe-inspiring: huge stained-glass windows, ceilings that seem to touch the sky, a peaceful quietness that invites you to sit and empty your mind. Imagine sitting alone in a church, repeating a simple prayer or letting your mind drift easily. There are no crowds to contend with, just you alone with your peaceful thoughts.

The process of prayer itself invites a calming of the body-&-mind. In addition to renewing our relationship with God, we quiet ourselves. And as we become calm and quiet we gain perspective on troubled times. Anyone who has successfully turned to prayer during a crisis knows this feeling. I am not advocating any religious undertaking. But if your spiritual practice includes prayer, I promise you that by letting yourself calmly, slowly, and meaningfully pray during a stressful time, you will literally loosen the tensions of the major muscles of the body and begin to reduce any current anxiety.

Other situations can produce this same sensation for you. When I sit by an open fire, watching the flames flickering, skipping from log to log, changing size and shape and color, I become pleasantly mesmerized by those flames. My worries and problems seem to drift away as my attention is consumed by the fire, its crackling sounds, its sweet smell.

Remember as a child lying in a field and watching the clouds slowly take shape? First comes a clear impression of Abraham Lincoln's face. Three or four minutes later it's a long train, slowly ambling across the sky. Without effort the clouds freely drift into pleasant patterns, allowing your eyes to relax their gaze.

Imagine fishermen sitting on the shore or in a boat, as still as their lines in the water, hour after hour. Their tranquil faces express a relaxed and easy quietness. Think of your own times of stillness and calm in the past. Have they ever come from rocking gently on the porch, back and forth, back and forth . . . no real effort, no pressures, just sitting and drifting? Or perhaps that peacefulness has come when you have risen early in the morning or stayed up alone late at night for some private time.

Focusing the Mind

When we focus on neutral or comforting thoughts and images, clear and measurable physiological changes take place in the body. As an experiment, read again the "Memories and Images" section you just read. This time, read slowly while you let yourself imagine each scene as I describe it. Try that now. If that experience begins to produce the Calming Response within you, here is what may be changing:

- Your oxygen consumption is decreasing.
- Your breathing is slowing.
- Your heart rate is decreasing.
- Your blood pressure is lessening.
- Your muscle tension is reducing.
- There is a growing sense of ease in your body and calmness in your mind.

You can contrast this with how you felt while you read earlier chapters in which I described anxiety-provoking times. *Our images have tremendous influence over our bodies.*

I am not describing to you some simplistic idea like "Just relax and you'll feel better." I am identifying the opposite and equally powerful capacity of the nervous system—the parasympathetic response, or Calming Response, which is essential to counterbalance the Emergency Response and all anxiety. And it is a capacity you already use. Anytime you feel comfortable and at ease, it is because of this Calming Response. Each time you fall asleep, it is because your Calming Response has quieted down the body-&-mind enough to allow sleep. What science has gradually discovered in the past thirty-five years is that we actually can activate the Calming Response through conscious effort. In the field of psychology, this discovery is as important as the achievement of NASA in placing the first humans on the moon. Our mental processes can alter the biochemistry of the body. An entirely new frontier is now open to us.

Finding Your Observer

Typically the responsibility for tensing and calming the body has been left to the unconscious mind. You probably are not aware of it when the muscles of your body become tense. I am not consciously aware of the number of muscles in my neck, my back, my arms, or my hands, which are contracting to help me write this sentence on my notepad. My unconscious does that detailed work for me so that I can consciously consider how to express my thoughts to you.

But muscle tension is a major component of anxiety and panic attacks, and if you are not aware of it during these times of difficulty, it can work against your progress. When you become anxious, your muscles automatically tense; that is the rule. The reverse is also true: when the muscles are not tensing, your mind has a chance to quiet down. To loosen and relax the muscles is an excellent method of activating the Calming Response. By the way, muscles don't actually "relax"; they are either not contracting or contracting to some degree. When I teach people calming techniques, I speak of "relaxing" the muscles to mean "letting go" of any muscle tension they notice. Unfortunately, most people who are afraid of a panic attack will physically tense their muscles and psychologically become anxious as a means of "remaining in control." They consider their tension to be a necessary way to stay on guard. But whenever you are highly tense and anxious, your ability to think logically is greatly diminished. The "solution" of bracing yourself contributes to the problem.

Set a goal to become skilled at consciously noticing and changing your muscle tension. Reducing that tension can automatically reduce anxiety and give you access to your Observer. Your mind starts to quiet all those useless negative thoughts so that you can concentrate objectively on the situation at hand. Any relaxation techniques and meditations taught these days actually increase your ability to think clearly, and therefore increase your self-control.

The Calming Response is part of your team that will help you master this anxiety problem. In this chapter we're going to build the components that will give you access to this valuable assistance. You'll learn about different breathing patterns and how they can support you. Then you'll have a chance to practice some formal relaxation and meditation techniques that give your body-&-mind an opportunity to feel mentally and physically quiet. You are working in this part of the book because you had difficulty getting away from your worries enough to apply some of the protocols in Part III. As you develop the skills to access your Calming Response, you'll find your Observer—the part of your mind that steps back, away from your struggle with anxiety. That ability will provide a foundation for changing your relationship with doubt and discomfort. Change it how? You are moving toward the capacity to notice your doubt and discomfort without having to fix them or remove them. As that ability strengthens, you can return to practicing the skills explained in Part III with renewed promise.

The Breath of Life

Breathing is an essential function of the body. With each inhalation, oxygen is delivered to the bronchial tubes of your lungs. Passing through the millions of tiny air sacs, the oxygen moves into your arteries, where it is captured by your blood cells. When blood circulates out of the lung area, it is bright red because of its high oxygen content. The oxygen-rich blood is pumped through the heart to all parts of the body. All the cells throughout the body then exchange their waste products for oxygen. The blood returning to the heart is duller in color because of its diminished oxygen content. The heart pumps the waste-filled blood back to the lungs. As you inhale more fresh air, a form of combustion takes place in which the blood cells absorb oxygen and release carbon dioxide. And the cycle begins again.

The respiratory system regulates breathing to maintain a balance of oxygen and carbon dioxide in the bloodstream. In normal circumstances, your rate of breathing is determined by the amount of carbon dioxide that must be expelled from your bloodstream and the amount of oxygen needed to satisfy the demands of your immediate activity.

Two Types of Breathing

Studies have revealed an important phenomenon that plays a significant role in mastering panic. During episodes of stress, people breathe more rapidly and, consequently, levels of carbon dioxide in the blood drop significantly. They also shift from breathing into the lower parts of their lungs to breathing into the upper parts. Figure 7 illustrates these two kinds of breathing, upper-chest (thoracic) and lower-chest (diaphragmatic). In upper-chest breathing the chest lifts upward and outward. The breathing is shallow and rapid. In lower-chest breathing, each inhalation is deeper and slower. Below the lungs is the diaphragm, a sheet-like muscle that separates the chest from the abdomen. When you fill your lower lungs with air, the lungs push down on the diaphragm and cause your abdominal region to protrude. Your stomach looks as though it is expanding and contracting with each diaphragmatic breath.

As research continues, we are learning more and more about the importance of these two breathing patterns. One study of 160 men and women found that those whose typical breathing pattern was slow and deep were more confident, emotionally stable, and physically and intellectually active. Those with a

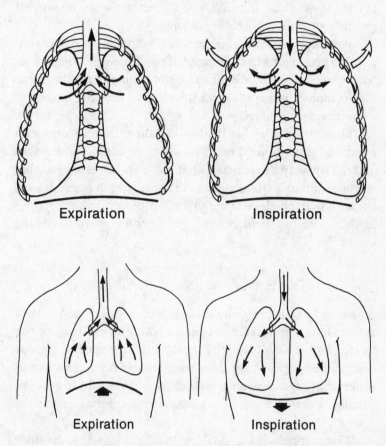

Figure 7. Two kinds of breathing, upper-chest (thoracic) above and lower-chest (diaphragmatic) below.

rapid and shallow habitual breathing pattern were more passive, dependent, fearful, and shy.

Rapid upper-chest breathing is a normal, brief response to any threatening or anxiety-provoking situation. It now appears that this kind of breathing is a stable, ongoing feature of people who are chronically anxious or phobic. In studies where chronically anxious subjects were specifically asked to begin breathing in their upper chest, they reported an increase in uncomfortable psychological and physical sensations.

Slow deep breathers, on the other hand, have a slower resting heart rate and a less "trigger-happy" Emergency Response. The habit of slow, easy, diaphragmatic breathing invites the Calming Response, promotes good health, and provides long-term protection for the heart.

These studies tell us that both short-term and long-term breathing patterns are directly related to psychological strength and the subjective experience of anxiety. By changing your habitual breathing pattern you can increase your defenses against panic. By changing your breathing pattern during an anxious episode you can help reverse your body's panic-provoking symptoms.

The Hyperventilation Syndrome

A change in your breathing should directly correspond to your activity level. For instance, if I am out biking for exercise, it won't be long before I am breathing rapidly from my upper chest. My body is now demanding more oxygen, and my metabolism is producing larger amounts of carbon dioxide, which must be exhaled. I can keep that breathing pattern up for as long as I'm biking.

What happens if I stop biking but force myself to continue breathing at that accelerated rate? I continue to exhale large quantities of carbon dioxide (CO_2), but I'm no longer depositing that amount of carbon dioxide into my bloodstream. Immediately my blood CO_2 level drops. When that takes place, CO_2 begins to leave my nerve cells, raising the pH level in the cells and making them more excitable. Because of this I may begin to feel nervous and jittery. Changes in the pH level remove calcium salts in my blood, which increases the excitability of my peripheral nerve endings, causing tingling around my mouth and fingers and toes. At the same time, this diminished level of CO_2

suppresses my Calming Response: my pupils dilate, my hands and feet begin to feel cold, my heart continues to race, lights seem brighter and sounds louder.

Simultaneously, the blood vessels in my brain constrict, which lowers the amount and the rate of oxygen transferred into those tissues. This produces most of my uncomfortable symptoms: dizziness, faintness, distortions in vision, difficulty concentrating, and a sense of separateness from my body (depersonalization). Most of these symptoms will develop within a minute of this type of breathing, called hyperventilation. If I slow my rate of breathing, all these changes will be reversed. Although uncomfortable, none of these short-term changes in the body's chemistry can cause lasting harm.

Often people who hyperventilate never realize they are doing so. They don't report that they are having a problem with their breathing. Instead, they complain of various specific or vague symptoms throughout their body. Specialist after specialist will search for thyroid, cardiac, gastrointestinal, respiratory, or central nervous system problems. The patient may be labeled anxious by the physician and referred to a mental-health professional, who can also fail to identify hyperventilation as the culprit. It is no surprise that people who are prone to hyperventilate are also anxious. But I would be anxious, too, if I continued to spontaneously experience such dramatic and undiagnosed symptoms!

Physical and Psychological Complaints
Caused by Hyperventilation

Cardiovascular

Uncomfortable awareness of the heart (palpitations)
Racing heart (tachycardia)

Heartburn

(continued on next page)

**Physical and Psychological Complaints
Caused by Hyperventilation** (continued)

Neurological

Dizziness and light-headedness
Poor concentration

Blurred vision
Numbness or tingling of
the mouth, hands, and feet

Gastrointestinal

Lump in the throat
Difficulty swallowing
Stomach pain

"Swallowing air"
Nausea

Musculoskeletal

Muscle pains
Shaking

Muscle spasms

Respiratory

Shortness of breath
"Asthma"

Chest pain
Choking sensation

General

Tension, anxiety
Fatigue, weakness

Poor sleep, nightmares
Sweating

Figure 8 illustrates how hyperventilation can be part of the vicious circle of panic. The process is as follows: (1) Any kind of emotional or physical disturbance can stimulate. (2) Hyperventilation, without the person's being consciously aware of the change. (3) The sensations of hyperventilation develop rapidly. (4) As soon as the person notices enough uncomfortable sensations. (5) He becomes panicky ("I can't breathe!" or "I'm going to faint!"). Before these thoughts are even completely registered in the mind, (6) the body has reacted to this interpretation with its Emergency Response (to face whatever is threatening the body). This further supports rapid upper-chest breathing and the cycle is re-created, with an increase in the number or intensity of sensations.

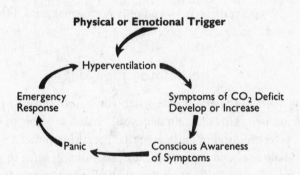

Figure 8. Hyperventilation in the cycle of panic.

Only minor degrees of hyperventilation are necessary to initiate its effects of increased heart rate, constriction of blood vessels, and a shifting of the acid-base balance in the blood toward alkalosis (a high pH level in the blood, causing light-headedness). If you want to see how quickly these changes occur, try this: breathe in and out as rapidly as you can for no more than fifteen seconds. Then sit back and notice the sensations in your body.

People who tend to hyperventilate appear to develop a general sensitivity to breathing patterns. The amount of carbon dioxide in their lungs at any time can change considerably relative to people who don't tend to overbreathe. Carbon dioxide levels drop markedly with any deep sigh, and recovery to normal levels takes longer. This instability, combined with the habit of upper-chest breathing, makes them even more susceptible to panic.

Once the problem is identified, recovery and control can be just as dramatic. In one study, more than one thousand patients diagnosed as hyperventilators were taught breathing and relaxation skills. For most of the patients, all hyperventilation sensations were gone within one to six months. Seventy-five percent were completely free of such problems at a twelve-month follow-up, and 20 percent experienced only occasional mild sensations, which were no longer troublesome.

The Foundation Skills

If you tend to hyperventilate when you get anxious or panicky there are two skills that can help you. First, learn how to breathe from your diaphragm and make that breathing pattern a part of your daily life. Old habits die hard, so you will have to work at this one. But by shifting to this slow, diaphragmatic breathing you will, over time, bring your blood carbon dioxide level back to a more stable position, and it will be less sensitive to brief respiratory changes. Second, become skilled at shifting your breathing pattern whenever you begin to feel panicky. Turn off the Emergency Response and encourage your body's Calming Response. When you calm down mentally, you can gain easy access to your Observer, so you can get perspective during anxious times. By calming the body and clearing the mind of negative comments, you will become mentally sharp and alert, ready to take care of yourself within seconds. Proper breathing can promote this shift.

All methods of eliciting the Calming Response can be assisted by one or both of the two types of breathing: what I call "natural" breathing and "deep" breathing. A simple exercise will teach you both of these breathing techniques.

1. Lie down on a rug or on your bed, with your legs relaxed and straight and your hands by your sides.

2. Let yourself breathe normal, easy breaths. Notice what part of your upper body rises and falls with each breath. Rest a hand on that spot. If that place is your chest, you are not taking full advantage of your lungs. If your stomach region (abdomen) is moving instead, you are doing fine.

3. If your hand is on your chest, place your other hand on your stomach region. Practice breathing into that area without producing a rise in the chest. If you need help to accomplish this, then consciously protrude your stomach region each time you inhale. By breathing into your lower lungs, you are using your respiratory system to its full potential. This is what I mean when I use the term *natural breathing:* gentle, slow, easy breathing into your lower lungs and not your upper chest. It is the method you should use throughout your normal daily activities.

4. Deep breathing is an extension of this normal process. With one hand on your chest and one on your abdomen, take a slow, deep breath, first filling your lower lungs, then your upper lungs. When you exhale, let your upper lungs go first (causing your upper hand to drop), then your lower lungs (causing your lower hand to drop). This deep breathing is used at the start of the Deep Muscle Relaxation exercise in the next section of this chapter and also in exercises later in the book.

5. Practice the natural breathing and the deep breathing several times, until you become familiar with each process. Remind yourself to practice the natural breathing technique often throughout each day. No matter how awkward it feels now, with practice it will eventually come naturally and automatically. Use the steps in the table below for guidance.

Natural Breathing

Give this exercise your full attention.

1. Gently and slowly inhale a normal amount of air, filling only your lower lungs.
2. Exhale easily.
3. Continue this slow, gentle breathing with a relaxed attitude, concentrating on filling only the lower lungs.

I'm going to teach you two formal methods of deep breathing: the Calming Breath and the Calming Counts. The first technique, the Calming Breath, takes about thirty seconds. To try it out, follow along with the instructions below.

The Calming Breath

1. Take a deep breath, filling first your lower lungs, then your upper lungs.
2. *Slowly* exhale, saying "relax" (or a similar word) under your breath.
3. Let your muscles go limp and warm; loosen your face and jaw muscles.
4. Remain in this "resting" position physically and mentally for about ten seconds, or for a couple of natural breaths.

The Calming Breath can be used any time you want to quiet down and access your Observer. If you need or want to have your eyes open because of your circumstances (you are driving a car or are with a group of people), feel free to do so. During your early weeks of learning, however, find safe opportunities to practice this exercise with your eyes closed. This will improve your body's chances of responding to your suggestions.

The second method of deep breathing is called Calming Counts. Read through these instructions before you try them out.

Calming Counts (First Practice)

- Sit comfortably.
- Take a nice, long, deep breath and exhale it *slowly* while saying the word "relax" under your breath.
- Let yourself take ten natural, easy breaths. Silently count each exhale, starting with "ten," until you reach "one."
- Through this whole time, permit your body-&-mind to respond to your invitation to relax. How might your body feel if it loosened its tensions? How might you feel emotionally? Invite yourself to be mentally quiet and physically loose.

In a moment, I'd like you to practice this process twice in a row, then make a small change the third time. Go ahead and begin your first practice now, and as you read the words again, let yourself read them slowly, as though you have shifted into a more gentle, quiet state. Let your natural breathing remain calm, gently inhaling into your abdomen.

Now, try it a second time, starting with that deep breath.

Now please try the experience a third time, this time taking *twenty* breaths and counting each exhalation, from "twenty" to "one." Practice this now.

As you finish the third time and before you become active again, take a moment to mentally scan your body. What do you notice? What has changed? How do you feel in general right now? If your body is feeling a pleasant kind of heaviness, lightness, or tingling, if you felt some of your muscles unwind, if your breathing seems calmer, then you are learning firsthand about the Calming Response.

Did you have trouble keeping track of the numbers? Did you become distracted by other thoughts? Did you make any worried, critical, or hopeless comments during the three practices? Did you become *more* anxious? Usually, the better able you are to passively concentrate on the counting, the calmer your body-&-mind become. The more you work at trying to concentrate (or trying to do it "right"), the harder this task becomes. So don't focus intently on how your breathing is changing, and don't evaluate how the exercise is progressing while you are in the middle of the experience. Simply let each exhale be a marker of the next number in your mind—inhale . . . exhale . . . "twenty" . . . inhale . . . exhale . . . "nineteen" . . . and so forth. When some other thought comes into your mind, gently dismiss it and return to the counting.

Once you have practiced this version a few times, use the instructions to continue to practice Calming Counts over the next few weeks.

Calming Counts

1. Sit comfortably.
2. Take a long, deep breath and exhale it slowly while saying the word "relax" under your breath.
3. Close your eyes, if you want.
4. Take ten natural, easy breaths. Count down with each exhale, starting with "ten."
5. During this time, remain mentally quiet.
6. When you reach "one," open your eyes again.

Calming Counts is another skill, like Calming Breath, which you should practice throughout your day, whether or not you are feeling tense. Such techniques, used several times each day, can help you reduce the buildup of normal, everyday tensions. If you begin to use them regularly during non-crisis times, you can create new pathways in the brain that promote mental calmness and muscle relaxation. Then, when you need this skill during a panic-provoking moment, it will almost be second nature. (I have written a transcript for a guided practice of these breathing skills. If you would like to record this guide in your own voice, the free transcript can be found at www.dontpaniclive.com. A pre-recorded version is also available.)

Your Observer and the Calming Response

Whenever your breathing settles down and your mind focuses on a few simple thoughts, you are inviting the Calming Response. During Calming Counts, when you notice your breathing just enough to count each exhalation, and notice and gently let go of any unnecessary comments, you are using your Observer. This exercise is an excellent way to teach yourself about your Observer and the Calming Response, as are Natural Breathing and the Calming Breath.

Remember that your primary goal is to find a long-lasting method for regaining control over panic. This is a one-step-at-a-time process. It is easiest to learn a new skill during low-anxiety times, when you are not feeling under stress. Once you have mastered the skill, then you can begin to apply it to the panic-provoking times. No one learns to type after they have been hired as a typist. And no one should expect these methods to work as effectively at first as they will after practice.

Releasing Tensions

If you have never had the opportunity to learn a formal method of producing the Calming Response, now is an excellent time to begin. In this section you will find a description of four protocols that each take about twenty minutes. You can choose one method to practice or experiment with each of them. If you have learned formal relaxation or meditation in the past, yet still have problems succeeding at some of the new techniques in Part III of this book, consider practicing them again. I suggest you practice daily for five weeks, and I have provided a form at the end of the chapter to help you track your commitment. Some of my clients who have successfully controlled panic attacks make formal relaxation or meditation time a continuing part of their daily activities, not just for five weeks. They consider it preventative medicine, just like getting regular exercise or eating a proper diet. Some follow the motto, "If you are too busy to meditate, you're too busy."

When you allow your muscles to rehearse again and again those contractions and relaxations, you are giving them a chance to create new pathways in the brain. Soon those pathways will be strong enough to give you much easier access to the Calming Response. Anyone who plays a musical instrument knows how much time and effort is required to learn those first hand movements. After persistent practice, those same movements come reflexively, without conscious thought. In that same way, by repeating any of the structured experiences in this chapter frequently enough, you have the chance to create new mental pathways leading to your Observer.

When you think about a situation related to your anxiety, mental images activate your major muscle groups into particular patterns of tension, as though bracing for a blow to the body. Dr. Edmund Jacobson was the first to propose that physical relaxation and anxiety are mutually exclusive. This means that if you learn how to recognize when your muscles are tense and can physically let go of that tension, then you will lower your emotional anxiety at that moment.

Dr. Jacobson developed a technique called Cue-Controlled Deep Muscle Relaxation (CC-DMR). It is based on well-researched and time-tested methods for training your body-&-mind to notice the subtle cues of muscle tension—and to release that tension. Some people find that a passive technique to quiet the mind and relax the body is more suited to their personal style than Cue-Controlled Deep Muscle Relaxation. You will have three choices if you prefer a technique of this nature. One is called Generalized Relaxation and Imagery, and the other two are forms of meditation practice, Concentration Meditation and Awareness Meditation. Any of these methods can be useful in learning the general skills of clearing your mind and calming your body.

Cue-Controlled Deep Muscle Relaxation (CC-DMR)

This three-phase exercise, which takes approximately twenty minutes, trains your body's large muscles to respond to the cues you give. You will begin by following nstructions to briefly tighten and then relax each of fourteen muscle groups. Then you will be guided through a full-body relaxation phase. During the last three minutes you will visualize yourself feeling safe and comfortable. Learning this particular technique is not essential to conquering panic. It is, however, one of the best ways to learn about your tension and how to alter it.

I suggest that my clients practice this exercise twice a day for one week, then once a day for the next four weeks. Why so often for so long? Because this is a straightforward, mechanical exercise that physically trains the muscles to release their tension. At certain intervals during the exercise, you are asked to repeat a cue word, such as "loosen" or "relax." It seems to take about five weeks of practice before the physical loosening of the muscles becomes associated with that cue word. You will be creating new "circuits" between your brain and your muscles, as I described in Chapter 10. Once the learning has taken place, the muscles will be prepared to release their tensions rapidly when you vocalize that cue word.

Remember, as you were learning the Calming Breath and Calming Counts, you were silently repeating the word "relax" as you exhaled. That should be the same word you use here. As you master CC-DMR over five weeks, the new circuits you develop will make the skills of the Calming Breath and Calming Counts much more powerful conveyors of your desire to quiet down.

If you want to record a copy of CC-DMR in your own voice, you will find a free transcript at www.dontpaniclive.com (space limits prevent me from offering these several transcripts within this book). A pre-recorded copy is also available.

Cue-Controlled Deep Muscle Relaxation is one method of developing the Calming Response by using your Observer. At the same time it helps prevent the tensions of the day from piling up. If you practice this method, you will notice Worried, Critical, or Hopeless Observer comments rising up from time to time during the twenty minutes. You should acknowledge and gently dismiss these negative comments. The final portion, in which you are instructed to "go to your safe place" in your mind, requires the greatest skill in passive concentration.

If you find that you have difficulty maintaining an easy, quiet concentration during that time, use the following One Hundred Counts exercise in place of your visual image. Begin counting silently with each exhalation, from "one hundred" to "one."

One Hundred Counts

1. Breathing in a relaxed, natural manner, count silently from one hundred to one, using each exhale as one count.
2. As you notice any other thoughts, easily let them go and return to your counting.
3. If you lose track of your counting, simply return to some number close to where you were.

Generalized Relaxation and Imagery

In Cue-Controlled Deep Muscle Relaxation, you rely on tensing the muscles first as a way to experience relaxation. As an option, or for an occasional change of pace, you may want to try the twenty-minute Generalized Relaxation and Imagery exercise. In this practice you will focus only on loosening—not tensing—your muscles. In addition, several new visual images are added to help you increase your sense of comfort and well-being as you enjoy peace and quiet.

You can record this exercise in your own voice by downloading the free transcript at www.dontpaniclive.com, or you can order a pre-recorded copy.

Meditation

Meditation is a family of mental exercises that generally involve sitting quietly and comfortably while focusing on some simple internal or external stimulus, such as a word, one's breathing pattern, or a visual object. In relaxation, you engage in a number of mental, and sometimes physical, activities. In meditation, you are physically still and have a much narrower focus of attention. After considering each method, you may prefer meditation instead of a relaxation technique as a way to release tensions.

There are a number of potential benefits to learning meditation. Meditation helps you to gain control of your physical tension by eliciting the Calming Response. Studies show that during meditation, as well as during relaxation, the heart rate and respiration rate slow down and blood pressure diminishes. Over time, meditators report feeling less daily anxiety, and they tend to recover more quickly after highly anxious times. Thus, meditation and relaxation provide similar gains for controlling physical tension.Meditation also offers the greatest distinct contribution to those who experience panic. Learning the skills of meditation can dramatically increase your ability to control your fearful thinking by teaching you new ways to respond to your automatic thoughts, emotions, and images.

If you are like the typical panic-prone person, you dwell on your worries, pay close attention to fearful thoughts, and respond emotionally to your negative images. Instead of being in control of these experiences, you are controlled by them. To learn to meditate is to learn how to step away from these experiences to become a detached, quiet observer of your thoughts, emotions, and images, as though you were watching them from the outside. Anyone who has experienced panic knows that the negative thinking during panic is so powerful that you can't simply say to yourself, "These thoughts are ridiculous. I am not about to die." That only invites a mental argument that increases panic: "Yes, I am about to die! My heart's racing a mile a minute. People die under this kind of stress." Any type of self-change strategy requires as a first step the skill of self-observation. To reduce your anxiety reaction and halt your negative thinking, you must be capable of stepping back from them far enough to put them in perspective. Meditation, as well as formal relaxation, gives you the foundation skills needed to gain that perspective, what I have been referring to in this book as your Observer.

There are two types of meditation to choose from. Since both accomplish similar goals, you can practice either or both of them. The first is concentration meditation.

Concentration Meditation

The four essential prerequisites for doing this meditation are (1) a quiet place, (2) a comfortable position, (3) an object to dwell on, and (4) a passive attitude. Just as with the relaxation techniques, you should use a quiet place to practice. Get comfortably seated and begin to invite a passive attitude within your mind, meaning that you don't need to worry about or become critical of distracting thoughts. Just note them, let them go, and return to the object you are dwelling on. The difference is that during meditation you select one object to focus on continuously during the twenty minutes. You may choose a word (such as "relax," "calm," "peace"), a religious phrase ("Let go and let God"), or a short sound (such as "ahh" or "omm"). Gently repeat that word or phrase silently at an easy pace. For instance, if it is a one-syllable sound, you might say it once on the inhale and once on the exhale. Or you may use your breathing pattern as the focus of your attention.

Both in meditation and in relaxation you are attempting to quiet your mind and to pay attention to only one thing at a time. An especially important skill to develop is that passive attitude. There should be no exertion involved in the meditation. Pay attention to the instructions, but don't struggle to achieve any goal. You don't have to work to create any images; you don't have to put any effort into feeling any sensations in your body. All you have to do is remain nonjudgmental and aware, be in a comfortable position, dwell on the phrase, and easily let go of any distracting thoughts until those twenty minutes are over. That is the passive attitude. And that is your Observer in its quietest form.

The following table is a modification of concentration meditation that uses One Hundred Counts, described on page 296. I have designed it especially for my panic-prone clients, because it offers two distinct advantages over traditional meditation. First, it gives you a stronger sense of being in control, since you must consciously keep track of the descending numbers. Second, it reduces the number of irrelevant thoughts that drift into your mind. This is most helpful during the times when you become flooded with Negative Observer comments. Meditation of One Hundred Counts gives you a specific and neutral task: to count with each exhale until you reach "one." This task will be in direct competition with your Negative Observer comments, therefore your mind will become less involved with such self-destructive thoughts.

Meditation of One Hundred Counts

1. Sit comfortably in a quiet place and let your eyes close.
2. Take a deep breath, exhale slowly and say "relax" silently.
3. Begin counting at "one hundred" while breathing naturally. Use each exhalation to mark the next number, until you reach "one."
4. If you lose track of your counting, simply return to some number close to where you were.
5. When other thoughts enter your mind, simply note them and let them go. Return to your focused counting.
6. When you reach "one," begin counting again at "one hundred."
7. When you reach "one" the second time, count forward with each exhale, from "one" to "ten." During this final ten-count sequence, suggest to yourself that when you open your eyes at "ten" you will feel alert and refreshed.

I have created a second modification of this technique called "Acoustic Meditation." It is an audio program that provides pleasant sounds, patterns, and rhythms to enhance your ability to concentrate. You can order a copy of this meditation at www.dontpaniclive.com.

Awareness Meditation

The second meditative technique is awareness meditation, also called mindfulness meditation. In concentration meditation, you use your Observer to attend to one object. You consider all other awareness as distractions and gently let them go. In awareness meditation, each new event that arises (including thoughts, images, and emotions), becomes the meditative object. Nothing that rises up independent of your direction is distraction. The only distraction is becoming involved in what you think, imagine, or feel, following it, embellishing, reacting, or becoming attracted to it instead of taking the stance of detached Observer of what you experience.

The process for awareness meditation is as follows. Find a quiet place to sit comfortably for twenty minutes. Begin by focusing on your natural breathing pattern. Mentally follow each gentle inhalation and exhalation, without judgment and without comment. (If you tend to become anxious when following your breath, you can focus on a single word or sound instead.) After a few minutes, allow your attention to shift easily among any perceptions that you notice rising up. As each new thought, image, or sensation registers in your mind, observe it in a detached manner. As you observe it, give that perception a simple label.

In the first few minutes of meditation you focus your awareness on each breath. By concentrating on something simple and internal, you quiet your busy mind. As you choose to loosen your attention away from your breathing, you will soon notice other perceptions. Perhaps you become aware of the tension you are holding in your forehead muscles. Without effort or struggle, subvocalize a name of the experience—perhaps "tension" or "forehead tension"—and continue observing. Within moments, your perception will shift. As your detached observing mind follows your awareness, maybe you take notice of a mental image of a man's face with the corners of his mouth turned downward. Do not become involved with the image; don't analyze its meaning or wonder why it appeared. Simply notice it and name it—"frown" or "man, sad face"—while you maintain your uncritical perspective. When you lose your detachment or become tangled up in emotions or focused on a decision, return your full concentration to your breathing pattern until you regain your detached Observer. Everyone gets caught up in their experiences, often dozens of times during each meditation. *Everyone. Dozens of times.* That is expected. Don't be self-critical if you continually drift off. In concentration meditation you merely relax, let go of the distraction, and focus back on your meditative word. In awareness meditation you relax, let go of any attachment you have to what you notice, and follow the flow of your perceptions from a distance. What you observe is not important. How often you get distracted is irrelevant. How you observe is the key: without evaluation and without involved comments. In those moments, you will find your Observer.

What You Can Learn from Meditation

You needn't become a skilled meditator to gain benefits from meditative practice. If you find that the two relaxation techniques are easier to follow, then choose one as a long-term method to relax your muscles and quiet your mind. However, if you practice meditation, even if only for a few weeks, you can learn a valuable skill that you can directly apply to controlling panic.

Consider that during anxiety attacks we become consumed by our momentary experience. We notice the unpleasant sensations in our body and become frightened by our interpretation of their meaning ("I'm going to faint," or "I won't be able to breathe"). We notice our surroundings and become frightened by how we interpret what we see ("There's no support here for me. This is a dangerous place right now"). We reinforce these sensations and thoughts by conjuring up terrifying images of ourselves not surviving the experience. Most of our thoughts, emotions, and images are out of proportion to reality. To gain control of these moments, we must become skilled at disengaging from our personal distortions. We need to step up on the platform of our Observer and comment on our experience without judgment. That's what meditation teaches. We will not develop this skill by waiting until our next panic to practice. By then it's too late, because panic has control. The best time to learn a basic skill is during non-anxious periods. That's the reason to meditate daily in a safe, private time and place. Then, we introduce that new Observer skill gradually, over time, into the problem situation.

Here are the valuable lessons you can glean from meditative practice:

1. Meditation is a form of relaxation training. You learn to sit comfortably and breathe in a calm, effortless way.

2. You learn to quiet your mind, to slow down the racing thoughts and to tune in to more subtle internal cues. You acquire the ability to self-observe.

3. You practice the skill of focusing your attention on one thing at a time and doing so in a relaxed, deliberate fashion. By reducing the number of thoughts and images that enter your mind during a brief period, you are able to think with greater clarity and simplicity about whatever task you wish to accomplish.

4. You master the ability to notice when your mind wanders from a task, to direct your mind back to the task, and to hold it there, at least for brief periods. At first there may be a longer interval between when your mind wanders and when you notice it. With continued practice, you learn to catch yourself closer and closer to the moment in which you lose track of your task.

5. Through meditation you desensitize yourself to whatever is on your mind. You are able to notice your personal fears, concerns, or worries and at the same time step back and become detached from them. In this manner you can learn about your problems instead of being consumed by them. That is your Observer.

6. If you regularly practice meditation and are able to feel more relaxed during that time, you gain the experience of mastery: Your voluntary actions produce pleasurable changes in your body-&-mind.

7. As you acquire the knowledge of how you feel when you are calm, then you can use that feeling as a reference point during your day. For instance, if you feel calm after meditation in the morning, you will have a greater chance of noticing the subtle cues of tension later in the day. In other words, meditation, as well as formal relaxation, helps you become more alert to what circumstances are stressful in your life. You then have time to

intervene in your circumstances before your tension builds to uncomfortable proportions.

8. In the upcoming two chapters you will learn the importance of noticing your thought process leading up to and during panic. You must develop the sensitivity (1) to "step back" and notice your Negative Observer thoughts, (2) to let those thoughts go and then, (3) to turn your attention to some specific support-ive tasks. That is no simple feat! By practicing meditation dur-ing a non-stressful time you practice those three steps without simultaneously struggling with the frightening experience of panic.

9. Some people attempt to overcome the anxious thoughts lead-ing up to panic by replacing them with positive thoughts. For instance, if they are thinking, "I'm about to lose control and go crazy," they will tell themselves, "No, I won't. I've never gone crazy before. I'll calm down soon." Sometimes this is a success-ful strategy. At other times, though, it can backfire by producing an internal quarrel. In arguments, we tend to "dig in" to de-fend our position, and that's what can happen here: the fearful thoughts only get stronger. If, instead, you can interrupt your fearful thoughts for a few seconds or a few minutes, you will be better able to introduce positive, supportive suggestions without risking that internal battle. The two meditative techniques in this chapter teach you this basic skill.

Which Method Is Best for You?

One essential purpose of practicing formal relaxation or medita-tion is to give your body-&-mind the peaceful rest that comes whenever you elicit your Observer and the Calming Response. By practicing one of these methods daily for five weeks, you learn how you feel when you calm down. You discover that you don't "lose control" as you let go of your tensions; you actually *gain* control. Choose whichever method interests you, then give yourself time to catch on to the technique.

I have outlined a number of benefits that can come from meditation. If you are a person who is plagued by many anxious thoughts, you will probably have an easier time with concentration meditation, rather than awareness meditation, because it provides you with a specific mental focus. Research suggests that people who experience predominantly physical symptoms of anxiety can diminish these tensions best through regular practice of active techniques such as Cue-Controlled Deep Muscle Relaxation. (Engaging in some form of regular physical exercise—such as walking, dancing, or active sports—can also help control anxiety that you express physically.) If you want a variety of suggestions during your relaxation practice and also want the pleasure of sitting quietly without having to move your muscle groups, then you will like Generalized Relaxation and Imagery. Even if you prefer one of the two formal relaxation methods, I suggest that you spend some time with meditative practice. Use meditation to teach yourself how to interrupt your intrusive Negative Observer thoughts, while you use relaxation to gain a sense of calmness.

Taking Conscious Control

Whichever approach you choose, your initial concentration will take serious commitment. Invest your time and don't be self-critical if you notice few immediate positive results. Use the time as practice, not as a test. When you finish any of the formal methods of accessing the Calming Response, do not immediately begin to evaluate how well or how poorly you performed. There are many variables that determine our responses to any particular exercise. For instance, on certain days when you are more anxious, your concentration may not be strong. Nonetheless, practicing the structured experience that day, difficult as it is, may give you greater benefits than if you had a "good" practice during a less pressured day. Any time you consciously choose to quiet your mind and relax your body, you are promoting your health.

Along with releasing tensions, all the structured exercises in this chapter will teach you how to rid yourself of unhelpful thoughts by first noticing them and then dropping them. Almost every time you practice one of the techniques, you will experience random thoughts floating up in your mind. The more you practice letting go of them, the greater skill you will develop, so that during actual problem times you will apply this new skill easily. If you get skilled at noticing a stray thought and letting it go during a Calming Counts practice or during formal meditation, then later, when you are entering a threatening situation, you will be disarming negative thoughts that produce tension within you. That is why you should never become discouraged about your progress on these techniques. The more difficulty you face while learning these skills, the better prepared you will be for the problem times. I cannot stress enough that repetitive practice will reward you tenfold over time. These methods need to become as automatic as your panic response is, because in the moment of panic you will want to focus on only a few simple thoughts. The more these skills become second nature to you, the better they will serve you during troubled times.

Consider that you are working to override the drama of panic. You cannot do that by generating a more powerful drama, since there is no more powerful drama than feeling you are losing control. Instead, offset that drama through the *repetition* of your calming skills. Repetition can trump drama; we have proven that to be true. We know from experience that if you structure a period of private time to quiet your mind and relax your body daily, panic will find less and less opportunity to intrude in your life. If you can combine a twenty-minute relaxation time with little thirty- to ninety-second mini-breaks of a Calming Breath or Calming Counts, you are building a strong foundation to support your efforts to control anxiety. The more rested you are physically and psychologically, the better protected you become.

Your First Important Steps

The best way to master a new skill is to break it down into learnable chunks. For instance, when you learn to type, you begin by repeatedly typing a few letters to master the proper finger movements. Again and again you repeat those patterns until your confidence builds. You then practice typing more letters in a row, then more complex sets of letters. You are instructed to type slowly at first so that you may concentrate better; speed will come later. The process then continues in gradual stages: two-letter words, three-letter words, five-letter words, phrases, and finally, full, punctuated sentences.

You need the same diligence and patience here. If you have never mastered a formal breathing skill or a relaxation or meditation technique, daily practice will build your skill and confidence. Slowly you will be better able to recognize when your mind and body are tense and when they are comfortable. Mastering any of the techniques in this chapter requires time. Remember when you first learned to ride a bike or to roller-skate? During your early attempts you probably said, "I'll never catch on. I'm so clumsy." But you persisted, and you learned.

So begin your daily practice today. You have two projects: your breathing skills and your formal relaxation or meditation. For the next two weeks, set a goal to stop for a moment *fifteen times each day* and do one of three tasks:

- Check if you are doing Natural Breathing (those gentle breaths in your belly),
- Take a Calming Breath, or
- Do Calming Counts

Post little reminders around the house, in your car, on your computer at the office, since fifteen times is about once every waking hour. Use Form 4 below to help you keep track of your progress.

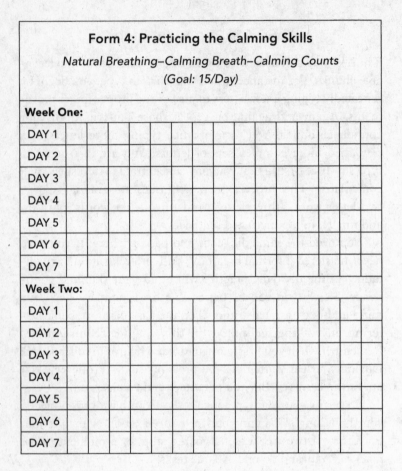

Form 4: Practicing the Calming Skills

Natural Breathing–Calming Breath–Calming Counts
(Goal: 15/Day)

Week One:

DAY 1														
DAY 2														
DAY 3														
DAY 4														
DAY 5														
DAY 6														
DAY 7														

Week Two:

DAY 1														
DAY 2														
DAY 3														
DAY 4														
DAY 5														
DAY 6														
DAY 7														

When you are ready to start your twenty-minute practice, then remember that during the first seven days you need to practice twice a day. This way you can intervene more powerfully into your unconscious pattern of daily tension. Then you can begin once-a-day practices. Form 5 can help you remember. You can also download all the forms in this book free from *www.dontpaniclive.com.*

Form 5: Practicing the Calming Skills CC-DMR–Generalized Relaxation–Meditation					
Day	Week One	Week Two	Week Three	Week Four	Week Five
Monday					
Tuesday					
Wednesday					
Thursday					
Friday					
Saturday					
Sunday					

You may feel these methods won't be powerful enough to affect your panic attacks, which you perceive as overwhelming. Let me say to you what I have said to my clients over the years: if you commit yourself to controlling anxiety attacks, you can do it. If you want to learn these new behaviors to conquer your anxiety attacks, then practice, practice, and practice some more. No one needs to be continually devastated by this problem.

CHAPTER 17

Take a New Stance:
Your Supportive Observer

For most of us, the world is full of decisions to be made, choices to consider, options to select. Every day we must discriminate dozens of times among an array of alternatives, from selecting the right combination of clothes in the morning, to choosing what to eat at each meal, to deciding which projects to tackle for the day. How do we make these decisions?

Within each of these arenas we develop, over time and through trial and error, our individual tastes. If I were to ask you to describe your favorite foods, the music you enjoy most, or your ideal vacation spot, you would probably describe the qualities you look for in making your choice. For instance, "I like a vacation spot with lots of sun but that's not too hot. Somewhere that isn't too crowded. And it would have to have water: either a pool, a lake, or the ocean." We discriminate among actual vacation spots on the basis of the characteristics we value.

Becoming aware of our general tastes and preferences makes each specific decision easier. I don't stand in the kitchen every morning, stupefied over whether I should have cereal, eggs, pancakes, French toast, oatmeal, granola, or just a glass of juice for breakfast. Since I am by now quite familiar with my likes and dislikes, I can choose in a few moments—usually oatmeal and coffee.

Filtering the Facts

It is the same with any of our decisions. The more we develop our sense of taste, our preferences, our values, our leanings, the less time we need to spend picking from an array of choices. Imagine how annoying it would be to spend a half hour reviewing each selection on a restaurant menu before picking an entrée. At some point we must trust our judgment. We must take a stand.

To make a decision we move through the same three stages I talked about in Chapter 15. First, we observe and register the information available to us. ("This menu has steak, pasta, and fish.") Second, we interpret that information on the basis of our knowledge, experience, and preferences. ("I had steak last night, and I'm not in the mood for pasta; I think I would like the stuffed flounder.") Finally, we take action that is based on our interpretation (we order the flounder). In other words, during the interpretation phase, we screen the information through our personal inclinations before we choose an action.

This process of discrimination doesn't always work in our favor. When the panic-prone person screens all collected information through the Worried Observer, the Hopeless Observer, and the Critical Observer, he reduces his options in a self-defeating manner. Each Negative Observer has its own special attitude about the world.

Here is a typical stance of the Worried Observer: "In all likelihood, things are going to turn out badly. I should be extremely careful before taking any action. What choice will keep me from experiencing any discomfort whatsoever? I must avoid problems. I need to feel completely comfortable. I'm willing to give up a lot if it will ensure that I'll feel safe. If I make the wrong choice, it could prove catastrophic."

The Hopeless Observer might filter all choices through this attitude: "I've always been uncomfortable in these situations, and I probably always will. Nothing's going to help. The same problems I have had in the past will continue tomorrow, next week, and next year. I'll never feel better. Things are just too difficult."

The Critical Observer may screen choices in this manner: "You'd better not make another mistake. The chances are that if you try anything new or bold, you'll screw it up and embarrass yourself again. You don't have what it takes to change. You are only good at failing."

Our minds are always interpreting and commenting on our experience of the world. To control panic you need to recognize your Negative Observer comments and interrupt them. If you don't interrupt these negative attitudes about yourself and the world, you will continue to feel controlled by panic. The negative attitudes will prevent you from taking successful action.

Let me give you a model with which to consider this idea, illustrated in Figures 9 and 10. During every moment of the waking day our minds observe the environment through our senses. Everything that we see, hear, touch, smell, and taste is a stimulus that is recorded by what I call our Observer. If our minds allowed this vast array of sensations to register fully in the brain, we could not make sense of the world. It would just be one confusing, overwhelming mess. Therefore, all stimuli that our Observer records go through an automatic, often unconscious, filtering process so that we can choose an appropriate response. That filter reduces the stimuli to a few simple ones, which we then interpret. On the basis of our interpretation of this filtered-down, simplified version of what we have observed, we decide how to respond (see Figure 9).

For instance, suppose you have decided to go out to lunch today. You drive into the parking lot of a restaurant. At that moment your Observer records all of your impressions: the color, size, and shape of the building, the number and kind of cars in the lot, and so forth. In the next instance you unconsciously filter all that data down to a few concepts and interpret them: "This is the restaurant that I wanted. It doesn't seem too crowded, either." You choose a response not on the basis of all the various stimuli, but on your filtered interpretation of them. You decide, "I'll eat here."

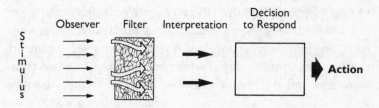

Figure 9. Simple decision-making process.

Now, suppose instead that sometime in the recent past you had a panic attack in a restaurant. Today you decide to go out to lunch with a friend. You drive up to the restaurant and observe the same stimuli as in the above example: the size, shape, and color of the building, the number of cars in the lot. Perhaps you even see people eating in booths by the window. Only this time you automatically and unconsciously filter all that identical data through your Worried Observer (see Figure 10). Now your interpretation completely changes: "This is a frightening scene! I'll be out of control here! It's not safe!" Now your decision changes, because our decisions are always based on our interpretation of the facts, not the facts themselves. This time you decide, "I'm going to become a nervous wreck if I stay here. I'd better avoid this place. How do I get out of here?"

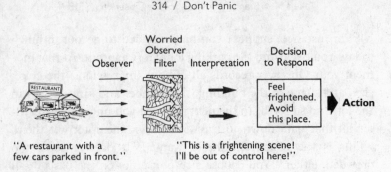

"A restaurant with a
few cars parked in front."

"This is a frightening scene!
I'll be out of control here!"

Figure 10. Decision making with Worried Observer filter.

This is why I say that to control panic you will have to learn to interrupt your Negative Observer comments. But, as they say in physics, nature abhors a vacuum. Your mind must always comment on your observations. If you interrupt worried comments during a panic-provoking moment but neglect to replace them with new and different comments, then those same negative thoughts will float back into your awareness. In other words, your mind will always use some filtering system; if you remove your Negative Observer filter you must replace it with a more beneficial one.

Your Supportive Observer

What qualities must this new filter have? During panic-provoking moments, the typical person needs several important resources:

1. *A sense of choice.* You need to feel free to move, free to change your direction. You want to know that you won't be trapped and won't be controlled by someone else or by some event. The greater the freedom you sense, the more willing you will be to stay in the scene.

2. *A sense of safety.* You need to feel protected from harm, safe to pursue your task. You need to feel secure in your surround-

ings. As you feel increasingly safe, you will feel more willing to remain involved in the event.

3. *A sense of support.* You need to feel stable and secure. You need to feel respected, nurtured, and cared for. You need to feel good about the choice you make. The more supported you feel, the easier it is to try new activities.

4. *A sense of courage.* You need to believe in yourself, have faith that you will make it through any difficulties. You need to trust in your own abilities, to believe that you can succeed but that you can also manage failure. The more courage you feel, the more power you have over your actions, even when you are scared.

In essence, you need to develop within you a new Supportive Observer—a supportive, courageous part of you that offers you a number of safe choices. Once you do this, you will gain a new perspective, one that will support your healthy, positive intentions and can come into play as a new filter during panicky times. To do so will take some time and much practice. One of the best ways to start is to regard your Supportive Observer as a new attitude that you can instill within yourself. That attitude has a particular manner of thinking about things. And it has a distinct voice.

Your Supportive Observer

- Reminds you of your freedoms and choices
- Gives you permission to feel safe
- Supports all your efforts
- Invites you to feel courageous
- Trusts you and lets you trust yourself
- Expects a positive future
- Points out your successes
- Looks around you for support
- Believes that you can change

- Knows that there is always more than one option in decision making
- Focuses more on solutions than on problems

"I Can . . . It's OK . . ."

The voice of the Negative Observer within us is usually harsh, dramatic, and extreme: "I can't let myself feel this way. This is going to be terrible. I'll be the laughingstock of the company. I'm being ridiculous. Nothing will work." Too often we believe that to control panic we must be strict and rigid with ourselves. We must suppress our uncomfortable sensations ("I can't let this anxiety continue"), contain our feelings ("I can't let anyone find out"), or limit our options ("A person should never walk out during a meeting"). This restrictive attitude ends up increasing panic's ability to control our lives. If the central fear in panic is the sense of feeling trapped, confined, or out of control, then the more messages we give ourselves that limit our options, the more we feel trapped by those limitations and the more discomfort we will feel.

Suppose I begin to feel a twinge of tension in my stomach just before I am to give a lecture, and I immediately think, "I can't let myself feel any anxiety." That thought alone is powerful enough to increase my anxiety. If instead I respond by saying, "I can handle a little anxiety here; it's normal to feel this way just before I begin talking," then I am not making myself feel trapped. By permitting the discomfort to exist, I am not supporting the increase of that discomfort.

See if these statements reflect any of your attitudes:

Typical Negative Observer Statements

- I can't let myself feel any anxiety. There is no acceptable level of anxiety.
- I can't handle these feelings.
- I can't let these symptoms continue.
- I can't let these symptoms increase.

- If I don't control these feelings they will run wild.
- I can't let anyone see that I'm anxious.
- I can't take the risk. I can only handle it this way! I can't change my routine.
- I've got to prove to myself that I'm better. (This is a test.)
- I know I'm going to get anxious as soon as I walk in there, and I don't want that.
- I must stay on guard at all times to feel safe.
- The only way to feel safe is to avoid all uncomfortable situations.

We put so many expectations and restrictions on our performance every time we attempt to actively engage in our world! It is no wonder that at the first sign of discomfort we tend to retreat, to avoid, or to run away. To face anxiety-provoking situations and succeed, we must give ourselves an easier task, one that allows for a greater number of acceptable options. As we adopt a more permissive, self-accepting attitude, we increase our sense of freedom and comfort.

Your Supportive Observer is permissive, accepting, and flexible. It gives you more freedom and more options. It is constantly working to keep you from feeling trapped, while simultaneously helping you move forward toward your goals. That is the gift of your Supportive Observer: it helps you feel safer while it helps you take action.

The Worried Observer mislabels your emotions. When you begin to feel uncomfortable sensations of anxiety, your Worried Observer filter says, "I'm terrified!" This knee-jerk reaction prevents you from noticing any gradual improvement in your ability to cope. Your Supportive Observer gives you time to notice your emotions. It helps you label feelings more realistically. When you notice some anxiety, it keeps those sensations in check: "I'm beginning to feel a little afraid right now." It can notice the subtle changes in your tension level—when it increases and when it decreases—without the high drama.

The Critical Observer reminds you of your flaws: "You're weak, and you're going to keep failing." Your Supportive Observe encourages you with what you *can* do: "Just focus on this single step. No matter what happens here, you can manage it. Then you can decide if you want to do anything else."

The Hopeless Observer underestimates your capacity to cope: "I can't. It's impossible." Your Supportive Observer says, "I'm not ready yet. Let me back up a step and try an easier task." It reminds you that you can be in control and that you can master your problems.

Two introductory phrases most aptly express your Supportive Observer attitude: "I can . . ." and "It's OK . . ." Listen to how your Supportive Observer might comment as you drive into that restaurant parking lot.

Well, here we are in the parking lot of the restaurant. I'm starting to feel nervous. Last time I ate out I had that panic attack . . . [pause to reflect]. I don't have to do this if I don't want to. It's OK to tell Susan that I'm just not feeling up to it. She really will understand. I don't have to keep this a secret from her . . . [pause to reflect]. I can also go inside and see how I do. I don't have to have the same reaction I had last time. I can feel safe in there. If I need to, I can get up and leave. Or, I can tell Susan that I'm nervous and get her support. There's no reason I have to stay through the whole meal if I don't want to. The worst that could happen is that I won't finish what's on my plate. I can handle that. So can Susan; I don't have to take care of her. In fact, she'll probably support me.

But I'm starting to breathe fast . . . This is *not* an emergency. It's OK to think about what I need right now . . . Let me just take a few Calming Breaths. I can let my muscles loosen a little. I can take time to calm down . . . [pause to reflect]. I think I'd like to go in, just to practice my skills of managing this scene. I really want to take this opportunity to practice. That's the only way I'll get better: by practicing my skills.

Notice how permissive that voice is. It knows that the more freedom you offer yourself, the better you will feel. It doesn't demand that you perform. You can stop whenever you want. It also reminds you that you can seek the support of others; you don't have to go through this all alone. In fact, you will find that when you give yourself permission to tell others, you will feel a great relief. However, the more you force yourself to contain all your thoughts and feelings, the more trapped you feel and the stronger your discomfort becomes.

Until you establish a sense of free choice within yourself, your primary need will be to escape. Once you establish that sense of freedom, you can consider moving closer to your goal. In this example of going to a restaurant, you will feel more comfortable about entering the restaurant since you tell yourself that you can confide in your supportive friend and you can leave if you need to. This is because the greater sense we have that we have the option to escape, the easier it is for us to enter. With every step forward, you offer yourself support and choice. The more you develop an attitude that permits you to have freedom of choice, the more you will be able to make healthy choices.

You can give yourself permission to reduce your discomfort. "This is not an emergency. It's OK to calm down a bit." It is also OK if you remain somewhat nervous. There is no reason you should feel perfectly calm while you are trying a new behavior. If you panicked in a restaurant recently, it is normal to feel uncomfortable the next time you enter. You can expect that and accept it, because eventually you won't be frightened. Eventually you will have managed this situation enough times to trust that you won't lose control and fall apart, go crazy, or humiliate yourself.

The most restricting attitude limits your behavior because of the possible opinions of others. ("I can't leave the restaurant . . .

because what would people think!") Developing your sense of self-esteem will improve your chances to use these kinds of messages effectively. ("I would leave the restaurant only as a way to increase my comfort. I deserve to feel comfort and a sense of freedom of movement when I go out to eat. That's more important than worrying about other people's opinions.")

Figure 11 illustrates how you can use your Supportive Observer to replace the Negative Observer filter. Through a permissive, supportive attitude about your actions, the general interpretation of the scene changes from "This is a frightening scene—I'll be out of control here," to "It's OK to take a chance here—this is a place to practice my skills." Instead of deciding to become nervous and run away, you can then decide to move ahead, one step at a time, just for practice.

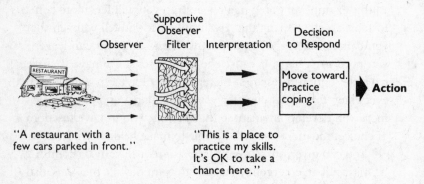

Figure 11. Decision making with Supportive Observer filter.

Here are more examples of this permissive attitude:

Supportive Observer Statements

- It's OK to take a chance here. This is a place to practice my skills.
- I can feel anxious and still perform my task.
- I don't have to let these feelings stop me.

- I can handle these sensations.
- I am free to come and go according to my comfort.
- I always have options, no matter what.
- Regardless of what I'm doing or where I'm going, I can have freedom of choice.
- This is not an emergency; I can think about what I need.
- I can be relaxed and in control at the same time.
- It's OK to feel safe here.
- I deserve to feel comfortable here.
- I can slow down and think.
- I can trust my body.
- As I learn to trust my body, I will have even more control of it.

Use Form 6 to write down some statements that can support you in your goal of controlling panic. Choose ones I've mentioned or design some of your own, then spend time reviewing them. You can even put them on your bathroom mirror or refrigerator. Practice using them each day and in any situation where you want to feel stronger. Begin to notice the difference between how you feel and act when you use the old self-critical or restrictive statements and when your attitude statements affirm your worth and your choices.

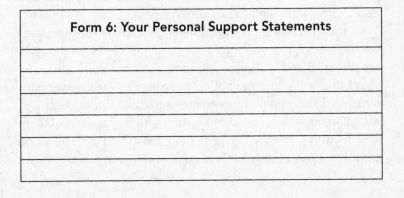

Form 6: Your Personal Support Statements

Stopping the Negative Observer

I have adapted this technique from a procedure, called thought stopping, which the field of behavioral psychology has applied for more than thirty years. Use it when you want to dispatch intruding thoughts quickly. This is how it goes.

To break a pattern of negative thoughts, first you must begin to notice the moments when you focus on Negative Observer comments. Often we are not aware that our minds are rushing through negative thoughts. As you begin to pay attention to the negative thoughts you will notice these moments more frequently.

The most straightforward way to stop your doubts and worries is to do it as quickly and powerfully as possible, before your mind is caught up in them. Once those worries strike—when you become aware of repetitive, unproductive, negative thoughts— mentally step back and observe them. Are your worries a signal of something you should pay attention to right now? Or are they just more noise in your day?

Ask yourself, "Are these thoughts helpful to me right now?" This is a great question; it will help you in a powerful way by confronting your automatic, negative thinking. Please don't ignore it! Simply by asking the question, you have momentarily interrupted your negative thinking, which is a good move. This is your Supportive Observer in action: it notices what you are thinking and decides if those thoughts are supporting you.

If the thoughts are not helpful—if they are noise—then consciously decide that you want to stop the racket. These thoughts are powerful and will draw you to them. They are drama, and your brain seeks out drama. Let your Supportive Observer reinforce your decision with statements such as, "I'm in control of my thoughts. I don't need to be run by these ideas. It's OK to stop focusing on this." Here is the most effective thing to do next: simply and gently let them go. You can keep noticing them, but stop attending to them as though they are relevant. That's the ideal response, and it should be your eventual goal (supported by Part III of this book). But if that's too hard for you right now, then you can use this technique.

You must make a firm decision of "not now." One way is to yell, "Stop!" inside your mind. I know that sounds like a silly thing to do. But yelling "Stop!" is a way to interrupt the drama of your worries. You fight fire with fire. It derails your current thought process and permits you to begin a new one.

If you need a little more stimulus to draw your attention, then wear a rubber band on your wrist. When you yell "Stop!" snap that rubber band at the same time. "Ouch!" Exactly! Now what are you paying attention to? That stinging wrist. For a split second you have left your worries and shifted to some other experience. You have created a space for a new focus of your attention.

Take advantage of that moment! Fill that space by practicing Calming Counts (the breathing technique of one deep breath and ten gentle breaths). Calming Counts will accomplish two important goals: They will interrupt your typical pattern of worry and you will perform a technique that actually calms down your body. You have to stop and think about how to do this highly specific breathing technique. You have to exhale all the way, take a deep breath, exhale again as slowly as possible, mentally repeating that cue word. Then you have to follow the next ten exhalations, counting each one, but counting backward. Boy, that's busy work! And that's exactly what we are looking for: something to keep your mind so busy that it doesn't drift back to your worries. Calming Counts takes about a minute and a half. That's a wedge of ninety seconds between you and your noisy worries.

Calming Counts can help reverse any anxiety that starts to build in response to your worried thoughts. As you get physically calmer and as time passes, you will gain perspective on your worries and have a much easier time resisting them.

Stopping the Negative Observer

Listen for your worried, critical, or hopeless thoughts.

↓

Decide that you want to stop them.
("Are these thoughts helping me?")

↓

Reinforce your decision through supportive comments.
("I can let go of these thoughts.")

↓

Mentally yell, "Stop!"
(Snap rubber band on wrist.)

↓

Begin the Calming Counts

Even if your negative thoughts return a minute later, you have briefly interrupted them. This is a method of bringing your Observer to the foreground during a time of trouble. Several minutes later you may want to interrupt those negative thoughts again with a second set of Calming Counts. Slowly, you will begin to mentally step back and see your worries from a new perspective. You will become less preoccupied, and your tension level will have a chance to decrease.

This technique is adaptable to many public situations. For instance, you can begin Calming Counts while waiting to give a speech. Instead of dwelling on negative thoughts such as, "Everyone will notice that my hands are shaking" or "I know I'm going to make a fool of myself," you can preoccupy your mind by keeping track of your counts.

This same negative thinking process takes place when we anticipate facing our fears. Imagine you plan to attend your neighbor's party tonight. You usually avoid such parties because you become nervous in groups. But this week you decide you will fight your fears by attending this gathering of friends. It is now 11:30 A.M. You notice that you have spent the last thirty minutes repeating useless Worried Observer comments silently in your mind: "I can't do this. I'll never last. What if I get trapped there? I don't want to get trapped. I can't go. I just can't handle it. I'll never last." At this moment your Observer breaks in.

OBSERVER: I keep repeating the same thoughts in my head about tonight. I'm scared. I've decided to go, but I keep thinking about how to avoid it.

SUPPORTIVE OBSERVER: These thoughts are only making me more scared. They aren't helpful. I can let them go.

ACTION: Mentally yells, "Stop!" Sits down for a minute and does ten Calming Counts.

OBSERVER: Now that I am quieter, I notice how tense my stomach is. I'm still scared.

SUPPORTIVE OBSERVER: Probably I'll be a little anxious all day. It's OK to be somewhat tense since I'm taking on a challenge tonight. I need to pace my day and keep myself fairly busy until it's time to get ready. That's a good way to take care of myself. I also want some support tonight so I don't feel like I'm going through this alone.

ACTION: Makes a list of a few worthwhile projects for the day that require some concentration. Shares concerns with a supportive person who will be attending the party. Monitors stomach tensions periodically through the day, using the Calming Breath to relax the stomach muscles when needed.

Notice what happened at the beginning of this example. I described your Observer as "breaking in" during your negative, obsessive thinking. This is probably something that already takes place within you now. You will become entangled in some negative thinking, then all of a sudden, some part of your mind will "step back" and comment on what you are doing. This is the moment you want to seize; this moment is the opportunity for change.

Begin to listen to your Observer rising up. When you notice it, *keep it!* Let yourself gather the facts of the moment objectively, then shift to some suggestion or plan that will take care of you and at the same time support your positive goals. If you begin criticizing yourself or making comments of hopelessness, simply notice them and then let them go. ("Thinking that thought isn't helpful to me right now.")

Interrupting the Pattern

Let's apply this concept of filters to the actual moment of panic. In a simple decision-making process, we move through three stages: (1) we observe relevant information, (2) we interpret that information, and (3) we choose an appropriate action (Figure 12). A panic attack occurs when that process becomes bogged down in the first two stages. Stage 1, we observe either our bodily sensations or our surroundings. Stage 2, using our Worried Observer filter, we interpret our sensations as "panic" or our surroundings as "dangerous." Then we turn back and observe our bodily sensations again.

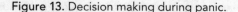

Observe Relevant Information ⟹ **Interpret Observations** ⟹ **Choose Appropriate Action**

Figure 12. Simple decision-making process.

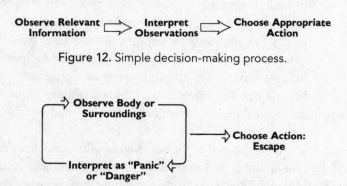

Figure 13. Decision making during panic.

We notice they are becoming increasingly uncomfortable. Next, we interpret these increased sensations as "panic," and so forth, in a continuing, escalating mental and physical crisis (Figure 13).

This is how we create panic. We become stuck at the point of focusing on and reinforcing the idea that a problem exists. Our mind gives one hundred percent of its attention to the problem and its potential repercussions instead of giving equal time to solutions. It fails to switch to Stage 3—choosing an appropriate action—until it has enlarged the problem to monumental proportions. By the time it shifts to the take-action stage, the only solution to this self-imposed, overwhelming crisis is to escape.

The essential first step in a panic-provoking moment is to interrupt that pattern. If you do not consciously interrupt the pattern, it will follow its normal course automatically, which typically concludes with you running away from some situation to avoid what you interpret to be your loss of control.

At some point during that process, you must stop long enough to notice what you are thinking. If you pay close attention, you will actually hear your Observer rise up spontaneously, reporting something about your current experience: "My heart's beating faster," or "I feel dizzy," or "I'm becoming afraid." Then your negative thoughts will follow: "Oh, no! What terrible thing is about to happen to me?" *That is the moment to interrupt the pattern.* Your job is to drive a wedge between your awareness of your discomfort and your continued negative, self-defeating thoughts.

Ideally, that's the time to notice your worried thoughts and let them go, and I encourage you to aim for that as your eventual goal. To let them go means to not embellish them or treat them as important. If that's not possible for you yet, then I offer the following structured response to the moment of panic, a way of directing your attention during panicky times. Consider it as a safety crutch that you use until you can apply the skills of Part III of this book.

Give your Observer some simple task to perform, one that requires no interpretations, no filters. By doing so you will be turning your attention away from your Worried Observer. You will also be inviting the Calming Response to begin quieting down your rising Emergency Response. There are a multitude of ways momentarily to disengage from this negative pattern and engage your Observer. Here is one major way: find something neutral or pleasant to do. I have listed a few examples below, some of which will sound silly, I'm sure. They all begin the same way.

Focusing Your Observer
During Anxious Times

OBSERVER: "I'm starting to panic."
WORRIED OBSERVER: "Oh, no!"
SUPPORTIVE OBSERVER: "This is not an emergency. I can care for myself by interrupting the pattern."

- Do a formal exercise, such as Calming Counts or a minute of repeating your meditative word with each breath.
- Take two or three Calming Breaths.
- If you are at your work desk, begin gently concentrating on a simple repetitive task. Don't bother trying to do the task well. Instead, concentrate on *doing it slowly*. For instance, open your file drawer and begin *slowly* counting the file folders. Or take out a piece of paper and write a few simple lists of any kind, *slowly* and methodically. If you are operating machinery, find some basic rhythm in your work and apply your breathing and counting to that rhythm.
- If you are walking down the street, begin *slowly* looking around while you continue to walk or as you stop and lean against a wall. Give yourself a minute or two of easy observing, such as deciding what color is predominant in the clothing of the people on that street or any other simple task. Or pace your walking with your breathing: two steps while inhaling, three steps while exhaling or any other easy rhythm.
- If you are in a restaurant or are a passenger in a vehicle, take out your wallet or purse and reorganize your pictures and cards. Or, pull out all your dollar bills and order them by serial numbers.
- If you are at home, peel an apple or orange *slowly* and with concentration. Watch the light mist spray out each time you

pull off a wedge of orange. Count each piece as it breaks off.
Or reorganize the books on one shelf. Or make up a bed
"army style," with attention to detail.

- If you are at a concert begin tracking the sounds of one
instrument or voice in detail. At a sporting event, track the
actions of a single player or official.

As I said, some of these suggestions do sound a little silly.
But the point is to do something that requires simple concentration, that has relatively little importance and that you can do
slowly and methodically. You will also need to pay enough attention to the task so you won't keep holding down that emergency
button. You are essentially calling "time out" on your negative
thoughts. You are taking a chunk of time to do nothing but concentrate on your Observer task. No checking back to monitor your
physical sensations, no evaluations of how poorly the interrup-
tion is working. Remember, this is Stage 1, pure observing. Any
negative interpretations ("This won't work") that intrude during this time—thirty seconds to several minutes—should be
gently dismissed.

Gaining control of these initial few moments will be a turning point. Once you have interrupted the pattern, even briefly,
your mind makes room for positive, supportive thoughts about
the problem. When you gain the edge of time, you gain perspective. Then, when you are ready, you can turn your Observer to
your physical sensations, your negative thoughts, or your environment.

Imagine that you are driving down the freeway when you
begin to feel anxious.

OBSERVER: I'm starting to get some panicky feelings.
WORRIED OBSERVER: Oh, no! I could kill someone!
SUPPORTIVE OBSERVER: I don't need to get all worked
up. This is not an emergency. I need to interrupt
the pattern.

ACTION: You decide to focus with your Observer. While continuing to attend to your driving skills, you decide to notice the license plate and color of each car that passes in the outside lane.

OBSERVER: [after a little time has passed] OK, here I am still driving the car. I've been paying attention to the license plates and car colors as a way of gaining perspective. I don't seem to be getting worse. I'm not losing control. What can I observe about my body? My heart isn't racing like it was. But I am squeezing the steering wheel really tightly with both hands, and my knuckles are white. I feel the knots in my shoulders. It feels like I am lifting my shoulders up to my ears.

SUPPORTIVE OBSERVER: I'm in full control of my driving even though I am nervous. I can loosen my grip and still have control of the wheel. I can loosen my shoulders. I'm OK.

ACTION: You take a deep breath, let out a sigh, loosen your hands on the wheel, and relax your shoulders. You concentrate on breathing calmly.

SUPPORTIVE OBSERVER: My driving skills are good right now. I think I began to panic when I read that sign saying, "Next exit 9 miles." I need to reassure myself.

ACTION: You continue your Supportive Observer comments. "I'm doing fine. I really caught myself early this time. I deserve a pat on the back. I can be nervous and still drive competently. I'll get where I'm going and back again."

The following table is a step-by-step summary of this process. Use it as a guide while you develop your ability to separate yourself from the messages of your three Negative Observers.

Taking Control of the Moment of Panic

1. Listen for your worried, critical, or hopeless thoughts about your body and your circumstances.
2. Interrupt this negative pattern by turning your attention to another task:

   • Take three Calming Breaths or do Calming Counts, or
   • Find some neutral or pleasant task to occupy your conscious thoughts

3. As you gain control of your thoughts and your breathing, observe your physical sensations, your negative comments, and your surroundings.
4. Answer the question, "How can I support myself right now?"
5. Take supportive action on the basis of your answer.

Inviting the Discomfort

As you know, I am encouraging you to work on these supportive skills so that you can return with renewed strength to the skills of Part III. At this stage, let me illustrate how a person can move from our current practice of accepting and tolerating sensations to the skills of Chapter 14, "Talk to Panic," where you encourage panic to "give me your best shot."

In Chapter 7 you read about Michelle R., who became so fearful of panic that she stopped driving and avoided staying home alone, taking walks, or shopping alone. After a few sessions she realized that she was contributing to her panic sensations by her Worried Observer thoughts. One morning, just prior to a business meeting, she caught herself asking questions such as, "What happens if you feel overwhelmed? Or if you get that panicky feeling?" Then she noticed that she immediately began to develop uncomfortable sensations, and moments later she produced an anxiety attack. At that moment she recognized that her fearful thoughts of panic can lead directly to her actual panic symptoms.

From this awareness, Michelle made rapid progress. Several weeks later she practiced driving alone and taking a few short walks. Her Worried Observer comments continued to hinder her:

> We agreed last week that I would return home from the session by driving on the freeway, and I did. Right before I got on the road I started to feel anxious. I thought, "What if I get a panic attack and I can't get off the highway?" I remained tense most of the drive and my hands were perspiring. But I started thinking that I had an option to continue or to stop, and I really wanted to continue. I felt good that I made the progress. The worst part was anticipating the drive, not the drive itself.

Notice how Michelle succeeds in switching from her Worried Observer comments to a Supportive Observer stance. Her toughest time is before starting the drive, because that's when her Worried Observer typically runs through a series of negative scenarios about the future. She worries about some catastrophic event that might take place if she keeps driving. Once she begins the drive she shifts into a permissive attitude, giving herself a choice. "It's OK to stop driving if I need to. Or I can choose to keep going if I want." By giving herself supportive options, she gains the confidence to continue. And she's able to follow through on her desire, which is to complete her task.

To fight panic paradoxically is to go against our basic instincts. I knew that Michelle needed to experience some success in managing her anxiety before she would be ready for my next instructions. Now that she was able to persist through mild discomfort and continued Worried Observer comments, I presented the idea of paradox: if you stop fighting panic, it will disappear. For the coming week I gave her the following instruction: "The next time you have fearful thoughts about panic, I want you to ask panic, at that very moment, to give you a full-blown panic attack. Tell panic to increase your heart rate, to cause you to become dizzy. Ask it to produce all your uncomfortable sensations."

As you can imagine, Michelle nervously laughed at my suggestion and questioned my seriousness. I explained the rationale behind this seemingly illogical advice. When we become afraid of discomfort we are supporting those same uncomfortable sensations by establishing an oppositional relationship. The more fearful we become, the stronger they grow. By reducing our fear we destroy this complementary relationship. We drain all the strength out of panic, because it requires our resistance in order to live.

In this same way, if you attempt to stop the sensations or try to fight them, you are simply supporting and prolonging them. If you practice a relaxation technique and then anxiously wait for it to reduce your discomfort, you will be disappointed. As I spelled out in Chapter 10, techniques will not conquer panic; attitude will.

Listen to Michelle's description of her experience the following week.

MICHELLE: I took a long walk on Saturday. First I walked to a shopping mall and bought a few things. That only took about half an hour, so I decided to walk down some residential streets. I felt a little panicky because there were no stores, and I didn't have my cell phone to turn to for help—unfamiliar territory. I took a few Calming Breaths and reassured myself. Again, I found that my anticipation of trouble caused me more problems than any actual symptoms.

DR. W.: What kind of thoughts did you have?

MICHELLE: I would think, "Here I am . . . People don't know me . . . What if I faint? . . . No one would help me . . . I could start feeling dizzy." Then I would remember to do my breathing exercise and to say some positive things to support myself.

Remember the exercise you told me about last week, "Ask panic to bring on the symptoms"? I was surprised that the thought came to mind, but at one point I said, "Go ahead, panic, increase my symptoms right now. Make me dizzy. Make me pass out on the sidewalk." And I sort of brought things back into perspective.

DR. W.: How do you mean "brought things back into perspective"?

MICHELLE: Well, for a few moments nothing happened. Then I said to myself, "No, you know you're not going to faint. You know this happens to you all the time. You can walk through this neighborhood, and you are going to feel good about that when you are done." It was easy after that.

Something else seemed to change after Saturday. I've noticed an overall difference in my attitude . . . about myself. I seem to be staying away from criticizing myself. I'm not as down on myself. It's as though I started accepting my symptoms and accepting myself. Then Tuesday I spent the night alone for the first time in ages. That went well, no problems.

Michelle's experience with paradox is typical. When you completely and honestly request panic to increase your uncomfortable sensations, those sensations will usually diminish instead. It is important, however, that you don't make a pseudo-request, such as, "I'm beginning to become anxious. Now, I'm going to ask panic to please increase this anxiety . . . but I hope it doesn't increase, because then I'll never be able to handle it. So this trick had better work soon!" By fearing an increase in uncomfortable sensations and trying to "trick" them into diminishing quickly, you fall back into the trap of opposing panic and thereby encouraging and supporting the discomfort.

Here is how we might analyze Michelle's activity that Saturday through the experience of her Observer.

OBSERVER: [While walking throughout the shopping mall] I'm enjoying myself here today. I'm surprised and I'm pleased. I've been here half an hour. I want to walk around for at least another hour to build my confidence. I could walk down some residential streets, but I might start getting nervous.

SUPPORTIVE OBSERVER: It's time for me to take a little bigger risk. I need the practice.

WORRIED OBSERVER: [While walking through the neighborhood] Here I am in a strange place. People don't know me. What if I faint? No one would help me. I could start feeling faint.

OBSERVER: I'm starting to get worried and panicky. I can feel my heart beating.

SUPPORTIVE OBSERVER: I can calm myself and feel reassured.

ACTION: Takes several slow, easy Calming Breaths. Tells herself, "This is not an emergency. It's OK to be somewhat anxious right now since I'm trying something new. I can be a little afraid and still take this walk. I am in control."

WORRIED OBSERVER: There aren't any stores around to turn to for help. I don't have my cell phone, in case I have a panic attack. Oh no, I'll never make it.

OBSERVER: I'm starting to get upset again.

SUPPORTIVE OBSERVER: I need to take care of myself right now. I'll try what Dr. Wilson suggested last week.

ACTION: Talks to panic: "Go ahead, panic: make me faint. Increase my symptoms right now. Make me dizzy. Make me pass out on the sidewalk." She stops walking and encourages panic to make her faint.

OBSERVER: [After a couple of minutes] No, I can tell that I'm not going to faint. My symptoms aren't increasing even though I'm begging panic to increase them.

SUPPORTIVE OBSERVER: I can walk through this neighborhood, and I'm going to feel good when I'm done. [Her discomfort diminishes, and she completes her walk.]

When you are controlled by panic you are run by the "I can'ts" of your Negative Observer voice: "I can't feel this way. I can't get anxious, because someone will notice. I can't handle this experience." As you begin to gain control over panic, you will notice that your voice shifts to the "It's OK; I can" of your Supportive Observer: "It's OK to feel this way. I can feel anxious and still perform my job. I can manage these symptoms." Gradually you can introduce the attitude from Chapter 10 of "I want to have these sensations to get better." Keep in mind that this shift represents more than just a difference in semantics—it reflects a new attitude. When you talk to panic you progress to the opposite end of the continuum. You invite panic to increase your discomfort. "I'd like you to make me perspire right now. I want you to increase all of these symptoms immediately." That's the ultimate form of paradox; it is opposite of logic. The continuum is illustrated in Figure 14.

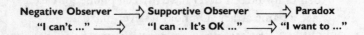

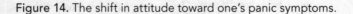

Figure 14. The shift in attitude toward one's panic symptoms.

Your Courageous Self

In a panic-prone situation, you will not remain in your Observer or Supportive Observer role the entire time. Your mind will float away into Worried, Critical, and Hopeless Observer comments.

You should expect that. As soon as you realize you are thinking negatively, interrupt that pattern. Return again to Observing, commenting with your Supportive Observer, and choosing an action. Whenever you feel in trouble, your first question should be, "How can I support myself right now?"

Here is one way to view this dynamic. Don't expect that you are going to completely eliminate the negative chatter with a replacement voice. Instead, consider that you are bringing up a parallel voice to support you and manage those negative thoughts. You will still hear that chatter, because part of your mind is still worried and believes you need to pay attention to its point of view. Your job is to incorporate that voice within your Supportive Observer comments and not let it be a competing voice that you must argue with. When you hear yourself say, "This is too frightening for me," you can respond by saying something similar to, "I understand how scared I am, and I'll be able to do this anyway." You will most likely continue to feel scared and comment about your fear, but you can base your actions on your commitment to your goals. That is courage: you feel frightened, you acknowledge those feelings, and you move ahead anyway. As long as you can find your Supportive Observer, panic will never consume your life again.

So practice all the skills within the chapters of Part IV. But plan on returning to Part III soon.

CHAPTER 18

Take the Hit

No more avoiding. No more backing away from discomfort. You have to step forward into anxiety and doubt to get stronger, and that time has come. But we are going to divide and conquer right now by helping you face only the physical sensations that scare you, not the events in which they occur. Once you master the skills of this chapter, then you'll be ready to return to the tasks within Part III. Or, if you want greater structure to help you face anxiety, then you can continue to Chapter 20.

But, First . . .

Let me remind you what you should have in place now, before you begin the practice exercises in this chapter.

- You learned about the benefits of backing away from your Negative Observer comments (Chapter 15).
- You began practicing formal relaxation or meditation, to learn what it feels like to quiet your mind and loosen your muscles and to train your body-&-mind to respond automatically to your cues (Chapter 16).

- You also began practicing your breathing skills fifteen times a day, to build up your ability to step away from your Negative Observer comments during stressful times (Chapter 16).
- And you identified Supportive Observer statements that can empower you as you face your doubt. These might include, "It's OK to take a chance here, I can handle these sensations, I don't have to let these feelings stop me" (Chapter 17).

All these skills—stepping away from your negative thoughts and not letting them dominate you, taking the edge off some of your tension through calming skills, and encouraging yourself to push into your fear—come into play here. It's like you are being propped up by the guidance of your Supportive Observer. You may sense this is a fragile and tentative support; that's fine. This chapter allows you to build the strength of your Supportive Observer, gain an alliance with the part of you that feels scared and practice pushing forward. You will be purposely trying out difficult exercises, but they last only two or three minutes. Most important, your efforts here give you a chance to develop faith in your new messages of, "I can handle these sensations."

Tolerate Sensations Outside Their Context

Panic tends to threaten you within one or more of four arenas of discomfort: your heart, your breathing, feeling dizzy or faint, and feeling detached from your body or surroundings. When you learn to face these sensations directly, when you discover they're uncomfortable but not dangerous, then they won't intimidate you anymore. The chart labeled "Practice Tolerating Sensations" on page 341 describes seven exercises that can provoke discomfort in any of us. Your job is to repeat them until they no longer intimidate you. Why go through such torture? When you later enter into a threatening situation and experience any of these sensations, you will have earned the right to say, "I've felt this many times before. I handled it then, and I can handle it now." You are going to want that belief, I promise you. To practice tolerating a racing heart and shortness of breath *while you are simultaneously carrying on a conversation with your boss* is pretty high up on the difficulty scale. It's much easier to isolate these sensations as you are learning to cope with them.

So, yes, I am asking you to do something that can make you quite uncomfortable. But do not skip over these exercises; they are your passage back into Part III, which, in turn, is your ticket to freedom. To get better, you need to purposely move toward two experiences—making yourself uncomfortable and being uncertain about what is going to happen next. Then you need to learn to tolerate that discomfort and doubt. There is no way around this; you have to go through it.

How to Take a Hit

Your job now is to teach yourself that you can handle the discomfort you have feared. That requires that you act courageously. You have to purposely become uncomfortable to learn that you can handle it. To create physical discomfort on purpose means you have to be willingly scared. That's no fun, but we're going to make this really short. Thirty seconds. One minute. Two minutes. And we're going to make this as simple a task as possible. You won't have to give a talk, or talk to a store clerk, or drive a car. All you have to do is sit there. And you can even do it with a friend.

What you will teach yourself now is that if you are willing to be uncomfortable, you can become comfortable again. What you will eventually learn, after a variety of practices within this book, is that during a panic attack, if you will decide in that moment to accept your doubt and allow yourself to feel anxious, you will end the panic. Essentially, if you do nothing, if you have as small a reaction as possible, you recover in the fastest possible time. You don't believe that yet. But you will. And you start by mastering this set of tasks.

How do you take a hit of anxiety? Willingly. How? By accepting it instead of resisting it.

Below is a description of the tasks, which are called interoceptive exposure, which means exposure to the sensations within your body. They are now a standard component of the cognitive-behavioral treatment of panic disorder.

Practice Tolerating Sensations

Task	Instructions	Possible Sensations
Staring	Stare at the dot in the middle of the grid on page 342. Or stare in a mirror at the bridge of your nose. Remain gazing, without moving your eyes, for 2 minutes.	Feeling detached, seeing spots, visual distortions
Any brisk exercise	Walk up and down stairs or use an aerobic exercise machine. Work long enough & hard enough to elevate your heart rate. Minimum 2 minutes.	Heart racing, sweating
Breath holding	Take a deep breath and hold it. 30 seconds.	Shortness of breath, heart racing
Breathe through straw	Breathe through a thin (cocktail) straw for one `then 2 minutes. Don't allow air through your nose.	Breathing difficulties, choking feelings

(continued on next page)

Practice Tolerating Sensations		
Task	Instructions	Possible Sensations
Shake head	Lower your head slightly and shake it from side to side for 30 seconds.	Dizziness, seeing spots
Head between knees	Place your head between your knees for 30 seconds, then quickly move to an upright position.	
Hyperventilate	Breathe deep and fast. Exhale with a lot of force. 1 minute.	

Staring Exercise Grid

Use a Coach

Ask a family member or friend to be your coach when you first begin these practices. A coach is like an externalized Supportive Observer.

Coaches can demonstrate how to do a practice and can practice with you in the beginning. And they should encourage you to practice frequently. But while you practice, including the thirty seconds after you stop, they should be silent, allowing you to concentrate inward.

Your coach should *not* reassure you that, "You're just fine, don't worry, I'm here." Why not? Because your objective is to expose yourself to discomfort and uncertainty. "Don't worry; I'll take care of you" is a reassurance that diminishes your doubt. Better is for your coach to say, "You're doing great; stay with it." After you practice each exercise (including that 30-second quiet period at the end), your coach can ask you two questions: "What are you feeling right now?" and "What are you thinking right now?"

Once you have mastered the procedures, then begin working alone so that you can develop your own internal Supportive Observer.

How to Practice

Start off by practicing each task three times. If it is easy for you—you feel comfortable or you feel uncomfortable but you rate your fear as low—then you "pass" that one and you can scratch that one off your list. You don't have to practice it anymore.

Just before you begin practice, fill out the first half of Form 7. Take a look at it now. Notice the phrase at the top of the Pre-exercise, "Once you notice the uncomfortable sensations." That needs to be your intention: to go get uncomfortable. When you imagine becoming uncomfortable staring in the mirror at your nose for two minutes, what are you afraid will happen? That you will start seeing spots floating around? That you will panic? Write your fearful prediction in that first blank (1). Estimate how likely it is that such an outcome will occur (2). Low, medium, or high likelihood? In the next two blanks, add what you think would be the best outcome (3) and how likely that is (4). I think the ideal outcome ought to be something close to, "I'm uncomfortable and OK with that."

For the tasks that do trouble you, commit to practicing them in sets of four repetitions, twice a day. Feel free to mix-and-match, switching among the tasks whenever you want. But master them all through practice; don't avoid the hard ones. Once you can consistently practice a task without becoming scared (a fear level of "low"), you can remove it from your list.

Form 7: Practice Tolerating Sensations		
Date:	**Exercise:**	
Intended Length:	**5. Actual Length:***	
Pre-Exercise	Once you notice the uncomfortable sensations . . .	
1. What outcome do you fear?		2. How likely?*
3. What is the best outcome?		4. How likely?*
Post-Exercise	6. Discomfort level*	7. Fear level*
8. What did you notice?		

* rate as "L" (Low), "M" (Medium), or "H" (High)

When you begin practicing any item, to the best of your ability practice for the length indicated. Attempt to remain as mentally quiet as you can. Simply follow the instructions and notice your experience.

During each practice, try to become as physically uncomfortable from the activity as you can tolerate. Your objective is to distinguish discomfort from fear, to learn that those uncomfortable sensations are nothing more than that: uncomfortable sensations. You don't go crazy, you don't have a stroke, you don't faint. Push yourself as hard as you can during these practices. Remember, your eventual goal is to not be intimidated by these sensations when you are out in the world. If you are timid with these practices, then you leave yourself vulnerable when you face them in the outside world. So don't distract yourself or use any other safety crutches. And push, push, push.

When the practice time ends, continue attending to your experience, while remaining mentally quiet, for at least another 30 seconds. Simply let time pass while maintaining attention to your sensations. Discover what happens. After you finish the practice, fill in on Form 7 how long you did the task in box 5, "Actual Length." Did you stay with the exercise to the end of your intended time, or did you get too scared and stop early? Then complete the rest of Form 7. In the first column of the Post-exercise section: How uncomfortable did you get? Fill in box 6 with low, medium, or high. Remember that your objective is to become uncomfortable. If an exercise doesn't cause at least medium discomfort, you can't benefit from it. In contrast, rate how scared you got by the discomfort in box 7. Quitting a practice prematurely or scoring medium or high on that fear scale—these are the indicators that you need to keep practicing this exercise. Jot down anything else you noticed about the experience in box 8. For instance, how did your prediction match the outcome? What are you beginning to notice? (You can print out multiple copies of Form 7 from www.dontpaniclive.com.)

Use Form 8 to track your practice. For the first three times you practice each task: if you complete it in the allotted time and with low fear (box 6 on Form 7), even with high discomfort level (box 7), then circle that number. If you circle 1, 2, and 3 (meaning the first three times you handled it with a low fear level), then you passed that task; you don't have to practice it again. The rest of the chart tracks two sets of four practices a day. Please note: You are practicing only eight tasks a day, four in the morning and four in the evening.

Task	Practice									
	DAY 1		DAY 2		DAY 3		DAY 4		DAY 5	
	AM	PM	AM	PM	AM	PM	AM	PM	AM	PM
STARING										
1 2 3 pass										
BRISK EX.										
1 2 3 pass										
BREATH HOLD										
1 2 3 pass										
STRAW										
1 2 3 pass										
SHAKE HEAD										
1 2 3 pass										
HEAD/KNEES										
1 2 3 pass										
HYPERVENT										
1 2 3 pass										

Form 8: Practice Tolerating Sensations

Keep your copies of Form 8 and see if you notice any patterns emerge. One pattern may be that even though you still predict a fearful outcome, after enough practices you start rating the likelihood of that problem as low. Simultaneously, you may notice that your "best" predicted outcome transforms into something similar to "I get uncomfortable and I'm OK with that," and you predict the likelihood of that as high.

CHAPTER 19

Face Panic

A Reminder

It's now time to head out into the world to practice your new skills. In this chapter, you'll learn how to set your long-term goals and your short-term tasks, and then learn ways to practice during each specific encounter with your fear. In previous chapters, I have emphasized breathing skills and formal relaxation techniques. These can play a significant role in your program. However, don't expect to stop panic only by using special breathing or relaxation skills. In the end, your strongest suit is to experience your negative sensations and learn to tolerate them. You can use such quieting skills in response to your uncomfortable physical sensations once they have started. You can also use them before uncomfortable sensations begin. But don't misdirect your attention toward strategies to avoid discomfort. Be willing to experience and to accept your doubt and distress.

Find a Supportive Ally

We humans are social beings. When it comes to solving problems, there is no benefit to working in isolation and secrecy. You will make your most productive advances when you support your own efforts, and when you spend time with others who support you. It is essential that you develop a Supportive Observer within you as you face panic. One way to encourage your Supportive Observer is to develop relationships with people who have supportive qualities.

Find at least one ally, someone who cares about your well-being and values your worth, someone who respects and supports your goals. In choosing supportive allies, look for the following traits: They remind you of your freedoms and choices. They give you permission to feel safe. They support all your efforts and invite you to feel confident. They trust you. They believe you can change, so they expect a positive future. They know there is always more than one option in any decision. They help you focus more on solutions than on problems. An ally may be your spouse, some other family member, a close friend, someone who has struggled with these problems before, or a trained health professional. Often a person is willing to support us but doesn't know the best way to go about it. Most likely you will have to explain to your allies how they can help. For instance, you might want them to read this book so that they can better understand the problems you face. Or you might need to explain how the Supportive Observer sounds, as described in Chapter 17.

This is not to imply that your allies must always be available to help you every step of the way. The most important role they play is to let you know you are not alone. When you know that someone in the world understands you, then you can feel you have a choice: you don't have to do this by yourself. You can feel safe: someone will be there to listen to you. You can feel supported: you don't have to be strong and independent one hundred percent of the time. And you can feel courage: with the support of your allies you can learn to face most threats.

When you have to completely depend on yourself, the pressures can be great. When you completely depend on someone else, you diminish your self-esteem and pride. But when you have someone in your life who is committed to a supportive relationship, then your personal power is greatly enhanced. Some days we are in no mood to pick ourselves up by the bootstraps, put on a smiling face, and meet the world head on. How nurturing it is to call someone and say, "Tell me everything's going to turn out OK." Hearing that supportive voice can virtually be a lifesaver. Over time, those supportive voices teach you how to talk to yourself in a sometimes gentle, sometimes firm voice that keeps this current problem in perspective as you explore solutions.

Face Panic Paradoxically

While you move forward toward your positive goals, assume that you will face panic along the way. When we set our sights on a challenging task we usually expect that we will work hard to achieve it. We make sacrifices and sometimes deny ourselves the easy way out of problems, because we know that is the price we must pay. Struggle and effort, then, are part and parcel of working toward a positive goal. There are no surprises in that logic.

The twist comes when we face our anxieties along the way. During these moments, the needed work is often to stop working so hard. That's what the strategies described in this book are for: to help you *not* struggle with panic. You can use any one of the several Calming Response skills while facing panic, but not so that you can better "fight" panic or "banish" panic at that moment. Instead, consider these skills as a way to a healthier perspective while panic tries to pick a fight with you. By changing your attitude toward panic, you withhold its nourishment. It dies off from lack of attention. Whenever you permit panic to exist while you keep moving toward your positive goals, you weaken panic's grip on your life.

This, then, is the paradox. You must always work actively toward your goals. However, when panic stands in your way, you take control of it by not pushing or struggling. Slow down long enough to regain control, then continue on your way.

Set Your Long-term Goals

Panic exerts a force over you. It attempts to push you into a corner where you feel trapped and afraid. To confront this force you must place some target in front of you, some positive goal to reach.

Creating your own goal will give you a clear sense of purpose. When you feel lost or confused, this goal can remind you of your positive direction. Let's decide to divide your goals into Long-term and Short-term. Long-term Goals represent your final desired outcome regarding your basic difficulties with anxiety. Short-term Goals focus your attention for only several days, weeks, or months. Often there are several Short-term Goals for each Long-term Goal.

Start by identifying your Long-term Goals. Take time to follow these instructions, writing down each of your answers. Use Form 9 to list all of the situations in which you have difficulty managing your anxiety and all the situations you avoid out of fear. Then, rewrite each item to create a positive Long-term Goal. On the following page is a sample form to help you get started.

Then, using Form 10, rank each Long-term Goal twice: from the least difficult to the most difficult; and from your highest priority to your lowest priority. This will help you figure out what to work on as you begin your practice. For instance, mastering restaurants may seem less difficult than learning to fly comfortably again. But if the job of your dreams requires occasional travel by plane, then you will rank flying higher on your priority list.

Sample Form 9: Listing Long-term Goals	
Events where I struggle or avoid	Positive Goal
Scared in restaurants	Feel safe in restaurants & enjoy meals with friends
Anxious on planes	Be able to regularly fly in a plane across country
Avoid parties or large groups	Feel in control at parties & enjoy myself without drinking alcohol
Afraid to drive far alone	Feel confident as I drive alone any distance I desire

Form 9: Listing Long-term Goals	
Events where I struggle or avoid	Positive Goal

IDENTIFYING YOUR LONG-TERM GOALS

1. List each situation when you have difficulty managing your anxiety and each situation you avoid out of fear.
2. Rewrite each item to create a positive Long-term Goal.
3. Rank each Long-term Goal twice:

   A. from least difficult to most difficult
   B. from highest priority to lowest priority

Form 10: Ranking Long-term Goals		
Long-term Goal	Ranking	
	Difficulty*	Priority†

* 1 = least difficult † = highest priority

Set Your Short-term Goals

Mastering panic also requires a smaller goal, which I call your Short-term Goal. This goal will be your immediate task that moves you closer to your Long-term Goal.

To understand the difference between a Long-term and a Short-term Goal, consider this example. Imagine that you are thirty years old and have worked as a transcriber for the past six years. After much soul-searching you feel a strong need to become more independent in your life's work. You decide to establish as your Long-term Goal greater job independence. Now what?

Your next step is to create a Short-term Plan that will help move you toward independence. You ask yourself, "What can I do today, this week, or this month about that goal?" The answer to this question is your Short-term Goal: "This month I will investigate what kinds of jobs might give me greater independence." This Short-term Goal now gives you a concrete and specific set of tasks to accomplish in the immediate future. Once you set your Short-term Goal, you always have some positive tasks to direct your actions.

Let's say that after a month of exploring options, you take another step closer to your goal: "I think there is room in this city for a digital transcribing service. With my experience I know what it takes to provide quality product to customers. I think I am capable of managing a small staff. But I don't know much about business." You set your next Short-term Goal: "I'll take a 'small business' course at night this fall at the technical college." Now you have a distinct focus. You must select the best course, register, buy the materials, attend class each week, complete your homework assignments, and so forth.

It is far easier to motivate yourself when your goal is almost within reach. Small decisions can now seem important, because they influence your immediate future goals. If you have difficulty applying yourself to your studies because owning your own business seems so far in the future, then you need to set a Short-term Goal closer to your reach: "By the end of this course I want to be able to say that I applied myself every week to complete the assignments of that week. Therefore, I will start by finishing my paper due this Friday."

This is the same process to use in overcoming panic. You might have the positive goal of "looking forward to the adventures of life without fearing panic." You will reach that goal by setting dozens of small goals, one after the other. As you accomplish one Short-term Goal you will set your sights on the next. Don't be in a rush to reach your Long-term Goal. By focusing too much of your attention on the distant future, you can feel demoralized and frustrated, as though you will never arrive at your destination. Instead, create images of your positive future, but work actively on accomplishing immediate tasks.

Here's how to establish Short-term Goals. From your Long-term Goal list, pick the two goals ranked least difficult and the two highest-priority goals. Using Form 11, for each of these Long-term Goals, list up to five Short-term Goals. These should be stated in positive terms that represent what you want to be able to do within several days or several weeks. Rank order each goal from the least difficult to the most difficult. If some of these goals seem daunting, then begin with the least difficult ones.

Setting Short-term Goals

1. From your Long-term Goal list, pick the two least difficult goals and the two highest-priority goals.
2. For each Long-term Goal, list up to five positive Short-term Goals—what you want to be able to do within several days or several weeks, stated in positive terms.
3. Rank your Short-term Goals from least difficult to most difficult

---

Form 11: Setting Short-term Goals for One Long-term Goal

Long-term Goal:

Short-term Goal	Rank*	Short-term Goal	Rank*

* 1 = least difficult

At any point in your day, you should be able to remind yourself of your Short-term Goal and create some task that moves you along. Do this not as a way to point out your failures or to criticize your weaknesses, but as a way to keep yourself motivated. Be careful of the Negative Observers, who are always just around the corner. The biggest troublemakers here are the Critical Observer and the Hopeless Observer.

You can spot the Critical Observer by its tendency to talk about the past: "I said on Monday that I was going to get out of the house for an hour's walk each day. Here it is Thursday, and I haven't done it yet. *I'm doing terribly! I'm so lazy!*" These last two sentences are not only useless, they are damaging to your self-esteem. When working on the task of conquering panic, set your Short-term Goals with your Supportive Observer. Often the words will be similar, but your tone will reflect a supportive, future-oriented attitude. The Supportive Observer isn't interested in dwelling on yesterday or even on the last hour. It pays attention to the present and the near future, in this manner: "On Monday I decided to walk an hour a day. Now it's Tuesday, and I haven't started yet. What do I need to do to take a walk today?" Not fulfilling your agreement yesterday is important to note. But you are not in control of yesterday; you are in control of today.

Again, paradox comes into play as you set your Short-term Goals and work toward them. The paradox is this: you should set a concrete, specific immediate goal, with every intent to fulfill that goal. At the same time, it does not matter whether you actually reach your goal in the way you expected. Let's say your Long-term Goal is to comfortably shop in stores again. You have taken a number of steps to prepare, such as practicing the Calming Breath a dozen times each day, spending quiet, meditative time for twenty minutes each day, and learning to give yourself Supportive Observer comments during stressful times. Now you decide to set a new Short-term Goal: "to walk around inside the mall today, looking in store windows with a friend, for thirty minutes." Once you commit yourself to that Short-term Goal, take as many steps toward that goal as you can manage. It is unimportant whether you accomplish that goal today, only that you give the goal your best shot. Set a Short-term Goal and move toward your distress and uncertainty to the best of your ability. Tomorrow you will simply review your learning from today and set a new Short-term Goal if needed.

We all deserve to feel a sense of pride and success. Don't rob yourself of those good feelings by labeling yourself as a failure when you don't accomplish a task. Do not define your personal success in terms of reaching your Short-term Goal. In conquering panic, you are successful anytime you are actively facing your distress as you move toward your goal, regardless of whether you reach it.

Create Short-term Tasks

In this planning stage, the third step is to identify specific actions that will move you from your abilities today to the abilities needed to reach your goals. After I show you two examples, you'll have a chance to generate your own on Form 12. Here is

Sample Form 12: Creating Short-term Tasks—Driving
Short-term Goal: *Comfortably drive a two-mile loop on roads around my house*
1. *Map out two-mile loop on roads around my house*
2. *With supportive person driving, ride as passenger on this loop, notice all chances to pull over, all gas stations, stores, & driveways that are accessible*
3. *Drive this loop during non-rush-hour time with supportive person as passenger*
4. *Drive this loop during rush-hour with supportive person as passenger*
5. *Drive this loop during non-rush-hour time with supportive person driving another car directly behind me*
6. *Drive this loop during non-rush-hour time with supportive person driving another car several cars behind me*
7. *Repeat step 5 during rush hour*
8. *Repeat step 6 during rush hour*
9. *Drive alone, with support person waiting at a point halfway along the route. Then have support person leave before me & wait for me at end of loop.*
10. *Drive entire loop alone while support person waits at finish*
11. *Drive entire loop alone while support person waits by telephone at another location*
12. *Repeat all these steps for different loops & for longer distances, until I can confidently drive any distance I desire*

an example of how you might generate a task list if you want to learn to drive comfortably again.

In order to look forward to the adventures of your life without fearing panic, one Short-term Goal must be to tolerate discomfort—from mild to moderate sensations of anxiety to a full-blown panic attack. If you can accept those sensations arising on occasion, and if you can trust in your ability to manage them, your fear of them will diminish.

Once you have set yourself this Short-term Goal of learning to tolerate that discomfort, you can establish Short-term tasks. Practicing the breathing and Calming Response exercises in this book is a good start. During this early stage of learning you can begin listening for your Negative Observer comments. Once you discover how your thoughts consistently reinforce your sense of fear, you can begin to practice Supportive Observer comments or other disruptive techniques. In this way you slowly chip away at panic.

Sample Form 12: Creating Short-term Tasks — Tolerating Discomfort

Short-term Goal: *Learn to Tolerate the Discomfort of Anxiety*

In the next five days, I will:

1. *Practice breathing skills ten times a day*

2. *Listen for & write down Negative Observer comments*

3. *Practice "Stopping the Negative Observer" daily*

4. *Practice Supportive Observer comments whenever anxious*

Make Your Tasks Reachable

When my first child was about fifteen months old, I watched in amazement as she grew in before my eyes. It seemed that each evening she showed me another "breakthrough" in her development.

One day she learned how to stack one peg on top of another. I watched her face contort as she tried to send messages of control to her hand, sliding the top peg around on the surface until it finally dropped into position. She probably expended as much mental energy as the Apollo astronauts did in making the first lunar landing. Then, the expression of glee spread across her face as she heard my hollers and applause.

As hard as it was for me to imagine, in another couple of years Joanna was talking in sentences, picking out her own clothes, and eating with a fork and spoon. And I was able to stop washing diapers. To me, there is nothing more remarkable than the physical and intellectual development that takes place between conception and a child's fifth birthday. From just two cells comes the most incredible creation ever contemplated.

Child development is a slow, step-by-step process. One way parents can negatively influence that process is by attempting to speed it up. A good parent is patient with the child, introducing just enough challenges to stimulate the child's growth, but not so much as to overwhelm. All good things come in time.

Many people who suffer from episodes of panic have been struggling for years and feel as though the struggles they face in the future will be too much to bear. To you I offer the same hopes and expectations parents have for their young children. The body is a phenomenal healing machine. It requires your faith, your commitment, your love, and your patience. With those qualities in place, it heals itself.

Just as your Critical Observer will focus on the past, your Hopeless Observer will think too far ahead. It looks at the distant goal and says, "I'll never get there. It is out of reach. I don't have what it takes to change." The Hopeless Observer has lost all curiosity; it never wonders about possibilities. Instead it uses your powerful skill of imagery to conjure up a picture of failure and concludes, "I can't."

Your Supportive Observer isn't wearing rose-colored glasses, looking through to impossible dreams, unrealistically imagining that you can do anything in the world. But its positive attitude is clearly distinct. The Hopeless Observer will look toward a distant goal and comment, "I can't." Your Supportive Observer will say, "I'm not ready for that, yet. What can I try now?"

These two comments may appear to be quite similar, but they aren't. When you say, "I can't," you are essentially closing the door on your ability to make a difference in your own life. When you say, "I'm not ready yet," you are presupposing that someday you will be ready. Your Supportive Observer keeps the door open for further growth and improvements, regardless of how long it takes.

There is always some step that is within your reach. If you feel incapable of accomplishing any of your tasks, you must create smaller and smaller steps until you find one to which you can say, "I wonder if I can do that? It seems within my reach." For instance, you don't begin learning public speaking skills by placing yourself at the podium in front of a thousand people. You learn by talking into a tape recorder and then listening to your voice, by telling more stories to your friends during dinner conversations or by imagining yourself comfortably addressing a small group of friends. If you fear panicking while you drive, the thought of taking a cross-country trip might be overwhelming. What can you imagine doing? Can you sit in the driver's seat of a car, with the ignition off, parked safely in the driveway, while you practice your Calming Response skills? If so, can you start the engine, back the car to the end of the driveway, then return it to its parked position, even if you feel somewhat anxious? Can you do that ten times? Once you feel in control of that step, can you drive around one block, with a supportive friend as a passenger? If not, practice driving to the corner and back. If that is not yet within your reach, let your friend drive the car to the corner, then exchange places and drive back yourself.

Regardless of what you fear, there is always a step small enough for you to take toward overcoming that fear. Whenever you run into difficulty, simply back up to a smaller step. The size of your step can never be too small. The Chinese philosopher Lao Tsu wrote in the sixth century B.C., "A tree as great as a man's embrace springs from a small shoot; a terrace nine stories high begins with a pile of earth; a journey of a thousand miles starts under one's feet."

Practice this step now by picking one of your Short-term Goals. Using Form 12, think of and write down a list of related tasks that gradually move you closer to accomplishing that Short-term Goal. The first item should be a low-risk experience that you can imagine accomplishing soon. Each successive item should include a little more risk-taking and should move you a little closer to your Short-term Goal.

Don't worry about creating the perfect schedule. Later, as you begin using this schedule, you will revise it based on your experience. Simply outline a stepwise approach to accomplishing your Short-term Goal.

Setting Tasks for Short-term Goal

For each Short-term Goal

1. Create a list of related tasks that gradually move you closer to accomplishing your Short-term Goal.
2. Review the list to ensure that

   A. The first item is the lowest-risk item on the list that you can imagine accomplishing soon.
   B. Each successive item includes a little more risk taking and moves you a little closer to your goal.

Face Your Tasks One at a Time

Some of my clients tell me that they feel most comfortable with activities if they can wait until the last moment to decide to par-

Form 12: Creating Short-term Tasks
TASK 1:
TASK 2:
TASK 3:
TASK 4:
TASK 5:
TASK 6:
TASK 7:

ticipate. Often this is true because these individuals let their negative images and thoughts run wild. If they commit themselves to an activity seven days in advance, they subject themselves to a week's worth of anxiety, fear, and grandiose negative fantasies. To take control of panic you must take control of planning your safe, enjoyable future. As you learn again that you can indeed plan activities in your life, then you will also be able to pleasantly dream about your future. Our plans and dreams fill us with the sense of hope that we each deserve, no matter what our past may have been.

For you, part of this planning must now include facing difficult situations. You won't be able to get around anxiety, you'll need to learn to go through it. Begin now by committing yourself to daily practice of facing your discomforts. Experience is the greatest teacher. All the reading and talking and analyzing and planning that you do will be worthless unless you translate them into action. You must act against your Negative Observer statements to overcome them. Don't let your fearful thoughts stop you. Don't wait for some magical day when you will rid yourself of panic without directly facing it. You must start doing things that you usually avoid, even if you have some sensations of anxiety. You must practice facing anxiety. So begin by dispensing with excuses that stall your progress. Chip away a little bit at your goal each day.

Now you are ready to begin working on the tasks you outlined above, while applying the knowledge and skills from all of the previous chapters. The stages of this step are: preparing for practice, beginning practice, responding to worried thoughts, responding to uncomfortable physical sensations, and ending the practice.

As you begin your practice, remember to face tasks one at a time.

- Don't look back to your last practice unless it is to remind you of your skills and capabilities.
- And don't look ahead as a way to remind yourself how far you have to go.
- Continue to practice a specific task until you feel relatively comfortable, then begin the next one. Never wait until you are completely comfortable.
- Don't measure your progress by how quickly you improve your skills. Measure your progress by how persistent you are in your determination to reach your Short-term and Long-term Goals. Shaping your positive attitude each day and developing a consistent schedule for practice—these two intentions will pay off with success.

Choosing a Short-term Goal

You will be practicing the Short-term Tasks listed under one or more Short-term Goals, so your first decision is to choose a beginning Short-term Goal. There are no rules for selecting the perfect Short-term Goal to work on; use your best judgment to pick one. You have ranked your Goals in two ways:

how difficult they seem and how important they are. Let those rankings help you make your decision. For instance, there may be a goal that is moderately hard on your difficulty list but is a high priority. Your desire to accomplish that goal may help motivate you to work on it now, even though there are easier items on the list.

You can certainly work on more than one Short-term Goal at a time. Perhaps you choose to focus both on the goal of driving comfortably to the mall and the goal of tolerating exercise that elevates your heart rate. You may have time in your week to practice driving skills every two days and practice cardiovascular workouts on the other days.

Preparing for Practice

There is a great array of options for practicing Short-term Tasks. In the beginning weeks, I suggest that you follow a structure similar to the one presented in this chapter. As you get more proficient at designing and implementing your practices, feel free to take short cuts. By the end, your practice can be as informal as this: "Hmm . . . I feel anxious about doing something like that. I think I'll try it!" One of my clients is working on construction in an office building. One day last month his coworker reported that one of the elevators had been temporarily stuck between floors for a few minutes. Upon hearing that, Alan became anxious and worried about getting stuck himself. Within a few minutes he excused himself, walked to the bank of elevators, and rode one to the top floor and back. He simply would not allow his fears to begin to take hold of him anymore.

Before practicing any Short-term Task that moves you closer to one of your Short-term Goals, consider each question in detail in the table below. Use Form 13 to write your answers down. You will benefit from making them concrete.

Planning Each Task

1. What is my Short-term Task?
2. When will I do this?
3. How long will I take?
4. What *worried* thoughts do I have about this Task?
5. What *self-critical* thoughts do I have about accomplishing this Task?
6. What *hopeless* thoughts do I have about this Task?
7. What can I say (in place of those negative thoughts) to support myself during this Task?
8. What support can I get from others? Who specifically?

Form 13: Planning Each Task		
1. Task:	2. When?	3. For How Long?
4. Worried Thoughts:		
5. Self-Critical Thoughts:		
6. Hopeless Thoughts:		
7. Supportive Thoughts:		
8. Support from Others:		

Deciding How Long to Practice

Whenever possible, practice your task for forty-five minutes to ninety minutes at a time. It is true that shorter practices also will help your confidence, and some types of practices can only last a few minutes (such as looking people in the eye and smiling as you go through a reception line). As you learned in Chapter 10, one of the most important purposes of task practice is to develop habituation: During prolonged exposure to an anxiety-provoking situation, intense anxiety gradually decreases. As your anxiety diminishes, you can think more clearly. In the future, when these situations occur again, you will react with some anxiety and some distress, but not with the terror that you once felt.

So when you can, design your sessions for this forty-five to ninety-minute length, which promotes habituation as well as confidence. You may have to repeat the same behavior several times. A goal of shopping for one hour may require a trip to the grocery store, then a walk next door to the pharmacy. And forty-five minutes will afford you lots of elevator rides! You may be surprised how much easier ride #15 will feel than ride #1 when you do them all in a row.

The definition of practice doesn't mean that you have to continually face your anxiety and doubt. For instance, you might enter the grocery store and stay only five minutes, then have to leave because of your distress level. For the next thirty minutes you may need to sit in your car, practicing your breathing skills to calm down enough to reenter the store. Then you enter the store for another ten minutes before finishing your practice. That equals forty-five minutes of practice—even though most of it was in the car—because all of that time you were working on facing your discomfort and tolerating it. Ninety minutes of aerobic exercise can mean that you run in place five minutes, then spend the next fifteen minutes calming yourself down if you get too scared, then another five minutes of aerobics and ten minutes of calming yourself, and so forth, until the time is up.

Creating Supportive Statements

Study your answers to questions 4, 5, and 6 in Form 13. These Negative Observer statements are the most likely to sabotage your efforts in the practice. Use them to design your supportive statements (question 7) on Form 13. Consider copying these positive statements on a card to support you during practice.

Turning Crutches into Springs

As you plan your practice, consider what you can do to support your commitment to venture into threatening arenas. For instance, you may feel safer—and therefore more committed—if you gather information about the setting or event. If you are attending a party, know what the appropriate attire will be. If you are driving a new route, check the map in advance or take the ride first as a passenger. If you are spending a night in an unfamiliar hotel, call ahead or go online to learn about their facilities. Bring along any props that can help you manage the situation. For instance, if you are practicing eating alone in a restaurant the first few times, you might carry a novel to read as you wait for your food. For a long drive, bring your favorite music or borrow a book-on-tape from the library. Decide if you would like one or more support persons to assist you in the practice. If so, choose people who believe in your worth and respect your efforts to improve yourself. They don't need an intimate knowledge of anxiety problems; in fact, they might be confused about the subject. But they do need to be willing to follow instructions! Tell support people exactly how you would like them to help. What should they say to you before and during the practice? What should they do?

I consider most of these options as "crutches." But as I described in Chapter 13, you can use crutches to help you spring forward into new practice territory. As you learn to manage that new scene through practice, then it is best to get rid of your crutches so that you can directly face your insecurity and learn to manage it.

Visualizing Success

Here is a brief visualization you can use during the few minutes just before you begin any Short-term Task practice. For instance, if you are about to enter the grocery store, you can practice this visualization while in your car at the store parking lot. It has two chief advantages. It draws your attention away from your Negative Observer comments and focuses on your desired outcome. And it reminds you of where you want to place your attention during the practice. It is not designed to predict how the event will turn out; it is meant to orient your positive attitude toward the task and help you remember your skills during a time when your mind tends to get distracted by worries. It only takes about three minutes.

Brief Visual Before Task Practice

Close your eyes and visualize yourself moving through your task. Let yourself experience two or three episodes when you have some typical discomfort. Then rehearse what coping skills you want to use to take care of yourself during that discomfort. Imagine those skills working successfully. Remind yourself of each of your supportive statements. Take a gentle, slow Calming Breath after saying each one, giving yourself time to believe it.

Beginning the Practice

Now you are ready to enter the troubling situation. Expect to respond naturally and easily to all that you encounter. Forget about yourself and pay attention to what you are presently perceiving with your senses: what you are seeing, hearing, touching, smelling, and maybe even what you are tasting. Use any of your skills to manage your thoughts and your uncomfortable physical sensations. Continue to encourage yourself and ask for any needed support from others.

At the end of Chapter 17 I presented a step-by-step summary called "Taking Control of the Moment of Panic." That design will help particularly when you suddenly notice the discomfort of panic. With this chapter you are planning anxiety-provoking activities, so you will be expecting to experience discomfort.

This allows you to respond to early difficulties before they build to a full-blown panic attack.

If you begin worried thoughts or if physical sensations begin to bother you, use the two approaches described below.

Responding to Worried Thoughts

The guidelines for handling worries during your task practice are simple: Notice your worried thoughts, choose to stop them, then apply skills that support your decision. Which skills or combination of skills you use will depend on your Short-term Task, the nature of your worries, and what has helped in the past. Sometimes you will need to explore several options before coming up with the most successful combination.

Responding to Worries

Notice your worried thoughts   "I'm working myself up."

↓

Choose to detach from them   "These thoughts aren't helpful. I can let them go."

↓

Take supportive action

START WITH
Take three Calming Breaths
OR
Do Calming Counts
THEN PRACTICE ANY OF THESE
Focus your attention back on your task
Supportive statements (Form 13, question 7)
Find something neutral or pleasant to do
Stopping the Negative Observer
(Chapter 17, page 324)

Responding to Uncomfortable Physical Sensations

As with your worries, the best approach to uncomfortable physical sensations is a simple one. First, mentally "step back" and notice the sensations without making worried comments. Second, reassure yourself: "It's OK for these sensations to exist right now. I can handle these feelings." Third, ask yourself: "What can I do to support myself right now?"

Choose among the supportive actions listed, depending on the nature of your discomfort, the circumstances, and what has helped you in the past. Here are some examples:

- You can assure yourself that you can manage your task while experiencing these sensations. You then can turn your attention away from yourself to the things around you. Involve yourself more actively in your surroundings (seek out a conversation or find something in your environment to study carefully) as a way to diminish your worried involvement in your body.
- You can use Calming Counts as a way to cope with your physical discomfort.
- You can tell a supportive person about what you are feeling and what you want to do to take care of yourself. You can let that person support your efforts.
- You can leave the situation for a brief period as a way to increase your comfort and control, then return to continue your practice.
- You can leave the situation and not return at this time. As you continue to practice your skills, over time you will learn to remain in the scene.

As you study the chart, you will notice how similar the actions are when your physical discomfort is your strongest concern. There is a primary difference. Can you notice it?

As you can see, there is one distinct difference in how you respond to worried thoughts and to physical sensations. As soon as you notice your worried thoughts, *choose to detach from them*. Reject the negative messages they are giving to your mind and body. The actions you then take support that decision. On the other hand, when you notice your physical sensations, you *choose to accept them*. This decision to accept your discomfort before trying to modify it is pivotal. Resisting your discomfort will only increase your discomfort. Most of the actions you can take are ways of loosening up your reaction, ways to help you not tense up *more* in response to noticing that you are tense.

Responding to Uncomfortable Physical Sensations

Notice your discomfort   "I'm feeling uncomfortable."

↓

Accept it   "That's OK. I can handle this."

↓

Take supportive action   PRACTICE ANY OF THESE
Focus your attention back on your task
Take three Calming Breaths
Do Calming Counts
Find something neutral or pleasant to do
Leave the situation and go to a "safe" place

Ending the Practice

Now is the time to support yourself for all your efforts. At the same time, review your practice session objectively. Assess what worked and what didn't. Use that information to plan your next practice.

Remember that you are successful every time you decide to practice, regardless of how long you are able to stay in that situation or how competent you feel during the event. There will be times when you feel embarrassed, clumsy, or awkward; those feelings are going to come with the territory, so you need to expect them and tolerate them. This is not a test of your ability to stop all sensations of discomfort. Nor is this a test of your progress. This, and every other thing you do, is an opportunity to practice your ability to support yourself. The more you practice supporting every effort and attempt, the stronger you will become and the more willing you will be to practice.

So listen for any harsh self-criticisms or discouraged thoughts after your practice: "I still get anxious. What's wrong with me! I'll never get better." Replace them with statements of support: "I'm working to change a lot of complex processes. I can't do it all at once. And I'm not trying to do it perfectly. One step at a time; I'm going to get there."

A Final Note

The trouble with our conscious mind is that it tries too hard.

Consider the performance of athletes. A professional athlete continually practices her drills and observes her techniques to improve her skill. But when it comes time to perform, the professional will stop paying attention to the details of her technique. Instead, she trusts that her instincts, her reflexes, and all her practice have sunk in. It does not mean that she knows that her instincts, reflexes, and practice will pay off with success.

What does trust mean? It means that she is willing to not know whether they will work, because she knows that the opposite—constant conscious monitoring—diminishes performance. She now looks outward, toward the game, toward the ball, toward the movements of other players. When she engages in the event she stops questioning or doubting her ability. She stops watching her style. In short, she asks her critical mind to quiet down so that her body-&-mind can do its work without disturbance.

Watch and listen to a professional musician performing a concert. He will play with abandonment, often without benefit of sheet music. All the necessary skills and memories flow out of the musician without a great deal of conscious effort. With effort, certainly, but not as much conscious effort. Professionals trust themselves at another level of being because they know that is the best way to support their efforts..

Too much conscious attention interferes with our performance, regardless of the task. The human body is the finest, most sophisticated, multisensory teaching machine in existence. Our conscious mind is but a minor player. To achieve our best performance we must not allow our conscious mind to become excessively involved in the process. True concentration is effortless, but the hardest job during concentration is to quiet the conscious mind.

All the dozens of ways in which I have approached the problem of panic pivot around the principle of trusting your body. Although many of the practice tasks I suggest in this book involve conscious thinking about each step, your final objective is to do very little conscious work. After you master the basic skills, practice keeping your mind off your body while you think very simply and slowly.

You will evolve beyond technique, all in good time. Your final goal can be to respond automatically and reflexively during times of trouble. You will know you have arrived when, one day, your conscious mind says, "Hey, what happened? I just handled that situation smoothly, and I didn't even know I was doing it."

CHAPTER 20

The Use of Medications

One of the most significant contributions of Western medicine has been the creation and use of medications to reduce patients' suffering. Medical researchers continue to investigate the benefits of medication for those with anxiety disorders. Current research efforts are focusing on all diagnostic categories: panic disorder and agoraphobia, social anxiety, simple phobias, obsessive-compulsive disorder, generalized anxiety disorder, and post–traumatic stress disorder.

In the following pages you will learn some specifics on the medications for three conditions: panic disorder, specific phobias, and social anxiety disorder. At the end of the chapter you'll find a chart of the medications used to treat all anxiety disorders in 2009. Please know that new medications are continually being tested for anxiety problems. For a full discussion of the medication currently used for treating anxiety disorders, and the benefits, doses, and side effects of each specific medication, go to the free self-help site www.dont paniclive.com.

Common Medications for Panic, Phobias, and Social Anxiety

Panic Attacks

For panic attacks, the greatest benefit that medications can provide is to enhance the patient's motivation and accelerate progress toward facing panic and all of its repercussions. For a drug to be helpful, it must assist in at least one of the two stages of panic. The first stage is anticipatory anxiety: all the uncomfortable physical sensations and negative thoughts that rise up as you anticipate facing panic. The second stage is the sensations of the panic attack itself. If a medication can specifically block panic, many patients no longer anticipate events with such anxiety and can overcome their phobias more quickly. Both current research and clinical experience suggest that certain medications may help reduce discomfort during one or both of these stages for some people. Another consideration is mood. If a patient is also depressed, which is common in 50 percent of people with panic disorder, then an antidepressant may help lift that mood.

The primary medications used today for panic disorder are several types of antidepressant and the benzodiazepines, which are sometimes used in combination with antidepressants.

The *selective serotonin reuptake inhibitors (SSRIs)* are the most commonly prescribed drugs for panic today and offer fewer side effects than the tricyclic antidepressants. These include fluoxetine (Prozac), fluvoxamine (Luvox), sertraline (Zoloft), paroxetine (Paxil), citalopram (Celexa), and escitalopram (Lexapro).

The *serotonin-norepinephrine reuptake inhibitors (SNRI)* venlafaxine (Effexor) and duloxetine (Cymbalta) have also been shown to help control panic attacks, as has the *mild tranquilizer* buspirone (BuSpar).

The most common *benzodiazepines* for panic attacks are alprazolam (Xanax), alprazolam XR (Xanax XR), and clonazepam (Klonopin). They block panic attacks quicker than the antidepressants, often in a week or two. They are also used as needed before a panic-provoking situation. They tend to have fewer side effects than antidepressants. However, they can cause withdrawal symptoms as you taper off them. Because alprazolam is quicker acting than clonazepam, its withdrawal effects can be stronger for some.

If you struggle in your willingness to face panic-provoking events, then the quick-acting nature of a benzodiazepine may prove helpful when taken as needed just before that panic-provoking event. It takes about 15 to 20 minutes to offer you its anxiety-reducing benefits. When it comes in tablet form and you place it under your tongue to dissolve (called sublingual), it can offer benefits within 5 to 8 minutes. Be ready for its bitter taste!

Clonazepam and the extended release (XR) formula of alprazolam last longer in the body than alprazolam. This allows you to dose twice a day for a full 24-hour coverage, while alprazolam requires four or five dosings for the same period. Some investigators believe they are a better choice than alprazolam during those times because their primary effects are not as strong and also wear off more slowly. While you are practicing the skills of facing your fears, if you notice the effects of a medication, you may tend to attribute your successes more to the medication than to your own efforts. Medications should serve as helpers to your own courage and skills and not get all the credit for good results. Because the effects of alprazolam XR and clonazepam's effects can be less noticeable, you will be more likely to say, "Hey, I did it!" instead of saying, "Boy, that drug really works well. Thank goodness it was there to save me!"

No reliable studies support the use of other minor tranquilizers such as oxazepam (Serax), chlordiazepoxide (Librium), or clorazepate (Tranxene), although these drugs may make the patient feel somewhat calmer.

Of the antidepressants, the *tricyclic antidepressant* drug imipramine (Tofranil) has the longest track record for treating panic attacks. Other tricyclic antidepressant drugs that can help control panic attacks are desipramine (Norpramin or Pertofrane), nortriptyline (Aventyl or Pamelor), amitriptyline (Elavil), doxepin (Sinequan or Adapin), trazodone (Desyrel), and clomipramine (Anafranil).

Monoamine oxidase inhibitors (MAOIs) are another family of antidepressants that manage the symptoms of panic. Research studies and extensive clinical experience show phenelzine (Nardil) as the preferred MAOI. Tranylcypromine (Parnate) is also sometimes effective. The antidepressants amoxapine (Asendin) and maprotiline (Ludiomil) are not generally effective for panic disorder. Bupropion (Wellbutrin) does not have enough evidence yet to verify its benefits.

If a physician recommends a combination of a benzodiazepine and an antidepressant, two approaches are possible. One is to take the antidepressant daily and use a benzodiazepine as needed to manage increased periods of anxiety or panic. Another method is to rely on the immediate effectiveness of the benzodiazepine during the first month or two of treatment with the antidepressant. As the primary effects of the antidepressant begin, after 4 to 8 weeks, the patient then slowly tapers off the benzodiazepine.

Specific Phobias

For people with specific phobias, medications can help reduce the tensions associated with entering the fearful situation. A patient can take a low dose of a *benzodiazepine* about one hour before exposure to the phobic stimulus to help reduce anticipatory anxiety. If this is not sufficient, the physician can prescribe a higher dose for the next time. A chemically dependent patient who is not currently abusing drugs might benefit from a benzodiazepine that is not attractive to drug abusers, such as oxazepam (Serax), or chlordiazepoxide (Librium).

It is important to note that medications are not a successful primary treatment of specific phobias. The treatment of choice involves many of the steps you have read about in this book. Consider medications only as an option to assist you in your efforts.

Social Anxiety Disorder

For social anxieties, medications can help diminish the tensions associated with entering the fearful situation, bring a racing heart and sweaty palms under control, and reduce some shyness. Physicians use several classes of medications that are beneficial, individually or in combination. These include the antidepressants, beta-blockers, and benzodiazepines.

The drugs with the longest history of use with social anxiety are the beta adrenergic blocking agents, also known as *beta-blockers*. The most commonly used are propranolol (Inderal) and atenolol (Tenormin). Surprisingly, controlled research studies have not supported the widespread anecdotal reports of success with beta-blockers. It's possible that their best use is for occasional mild social anxieties associated with performance. The high potency *benzodiazepines* clonazepam and alprazolam may also be effective. A combination of a beta-blocker and low dosages of clonazepam or alprazolam could be best for some individuals.

Current research suggests that the MAOIs, especially phenelzine, are most highly effective medications for treating people with the more generalized form of social anxiety. Occasionally, however, a person with social anxiety can experience an exaggerated response to an MAOI and become too talkative, outgoing, or socially uninhibited. In that case the prescribing physician will lower the medication dosage or stop it altogether.

One approach to drug treatment that experts recommend for social fears is to begin by taking a medication only as needed. If patients are anxious only about specific events and if they experience primarily physical discomfort (sweating, racing heart, etc.), then about one hour before the event, they can take propranolol or atenolol. Propranolol seems to work better for occasional problems, while atenolol may work better for continued problems. If their symptoms are more cognitive (they worry about their performance or the judgment of others), then they can take alprazolam one hour before the event. If they have a mix of these symptoms then a combination of these medications may be more helpful. Benefits of these drugs should last about four hours.

If the social anxiety is more general, unpredictable, and widespread, then the physician may recommend the SNRI venlafaxine, an MAOI such as phenelzine, or an SSRI such as sertraline. Keep in mind that these medications take several weeks to work. Bupropion (Wellbutrin) does not have enough evidence yet to verify its effectiveness for social anxiety disorder.

Enhancing Learning During Treatment

In behavior therapy, one central approach is to reduce fear by repeatedly pairing the feared stimulus with either relaxation or some other response that is counter to the fear. This can sometimes seem intimidating to patients. In a novel approach to treating anxiety, researchers are exploring the use of *d-cycloserine (DCS),* an antibiotic, to enhance learning and memory during behavioral treatment. It is possible that DCS may reorder connections between perception and the fear response. Early studies indicate that, at least at the beginning of behavioral treatment, patients taking DCS are more motivated to remain in therapy long enough to start noticing benefits.

Guidelines for Medication Use

If you would like to consider medication as a form of treatment for your anxiety symptoms, here are a few points that may make the process easier.

Begin by Obtaining an Accurate Diagnosis

If you are having anxiety symptoms, follow the instructions outlined in Chapter 2 to determine first if there is any physical cause. If your physician makes no physical diagnosis, he or she should refer you for an evaluation by a licensed mental health professional who specializes in anxiety disorders. Once you receive a diagnosis, your options for medications will be clearer.

There Is No Magic Pill

Complex problems do not have simple solutions, although many people will look for a quick cure and a magic pill. If they can find a sympathetic physician, they will begin a regimen of medications as their only means of removing all discomfort. Unfortunately, reports in the media that present a limited analysis of a complex problem reinforce the belief that medications are the only answer. By deciding to believe that they have an uncontrollable physical disorder or brain disorder, some patients surrender themselves to anxiety and panic. In the process, they lose self-esteem, determination, and the willingness to trust in the healing power of their bodies and minds. They remain dependent on medications, physicians, friends, and family as they continue to limit their personal freedom.

Among clinicians who specialize in anxiety disorders, there is general agreement that medications can be beneficial for some anxious patients when used in conjunction with a treatment approach similar to the one outlined in this book—one that directs you toward altering your negative thoughts and encouraging your ability to face those situations that you fear. Although we base treatment on the specific problems and resources of each patient, the key to success lies in your sense of personal ability to face the fearful situations and master discomfort and doubt. All professional interventions, whether in the form of individual therapy, group therapy, medication, behavioral techniques, or self-help, should have but one purpose: to stabilize your belief that *you are able to exert personal control over your body and your life.*

Take medications within this context. Often medicines can be a beneficial short-term crutch to help while you heal yourself. They do not heal you any more than a cast heals a broken leg. The body heals itself of many problems, given the proper support. For some people, medications offer a good long-term support for a disorder that can be chronic and cyclical in nature. Without medications, they seem to relapse into troubling symptoms.

Don't Suffer Needlessly to Prove You Are "Strong"

Some people believe that medications are for "weak" people, and they don't want to be "dependent." These people tend to make three mistakes. They avoid taking medications at all, when medications could play an appropriate and significant part in their self-help program. Or they underdose the medication they are taking, falsely believing that "less is better." Or they prematurely decelerate from a medication that is currently helping them. Medications can be effective, and they can be appropriate for you, depending on your problem. There is a specific dose that will be best for you that your physician will help identify. And there is justification for some people to remain on medication even for years if the side effects are not troubling them, if they are not trying to get pregnant, and if the symptoms tend to return with a vengeance when they experiment with withdrawing from the medication during cognitive-behavioral therapy.

If You Decide to Use a Medication, Give It a Fair Trial

To evaluate the benefit of a medication, you must give it enough time to provide its therapeutic effect. Work with your physician, especially in the early weeks of your medication trial, to adjust the dose and to relieve any worries you might have. Most physicians will initiate any of these drugs at a low dose and then slowly increase the dose, according to your response. You will need a trial of several weeks at full dose to determine the benefits.

Be Willing to Tolerate Some Side Effects

Side effects are unwanted psychological or physical changes that typically are not directly related to a medication's capability to treat a disorder. Most medications have some kind of side effects. Most will be minor symptoms that may be bothersome to you but do not require medical attention. These side effects may also diminish or end in a few days or weeks as your body adjusts to the medication. Rarely, they can be serious. Before starting a medication, ask your physician about possible side effects: what can you expect, what might diminish over time, and what needs his or her attention. Report any persistent or unexpected side effects to your prescribing physician.

I suggest that you educate yourself about the possible side effects, not because these medications are more powerful or more harmful than other drugs, but so that you can tolerate some of the minor symptoms instead of being scared off by them. For instance, the symptoms of dry mouth, blurred near vision, constipation, and difficulty with urination are common side effects of a number of drugs, especially the tricyclic antidepressants. Often side effects diminish in a few weeks as your body adjusts or when you reduce the dosage. In the meantime, your prescribing physician may suggest ways of relieving the discomfort. You can relieve a dry mouth by frequent rinsing or by sucking on hard candy or chewing gum. Blurred vision may clear up in a couple of weeks. If not, a new eyeglass prescription can help. You can counterbalance mild constipation by increasing your intake of bran, fluids (at least six glasses a day), and fresh fruits and vegetables. A laxative may also help. To assist with problems urinating, your doctor may prescribe bethanecol (Urecholine).

Another possible side effect is postural hypotension, also called orthostatic hypotension. This is a lowering of the blood pressure as you stand up from a sitting or lying position or after prolonged standing. This disequilibrium can cause sensations of dizziness or light-headedness and sometimes fatigue, especially in the morning when you get out of bed. These are signs that your circulatory system needs a little more time to distribute blood equally throughout your body. You may also notice an increase in your heart rate (tachycardia or palpitations) to compensate for this brief hypotension. When this side effect is mild, doctors advise that you get out of bed more slowly in the morning, sitting at the side of the bed for a full minute before standing, and that you also take your time rising from a seated position during the day. If you feel dizzy, give your body a minute to adjust to the standing position. You may also benefit from increasing your salt and fluid intake or wearing constrictive support hose.

Here are some ways to deal with a few other common side effects. Some medications have a sedating effect, making you drowsy. Physicians suggest that you take those medications close to bedtime if medically appropriate. On the other hand, if a drug causes you to have difficulty sleeping, they may suggest taking the medicine in the morning. As an alternative for either problem, you may need to lower the dose or change medications. For increased sweating, be sure you increase your fluid intake in warm weather to avoid dehydration. For weight gain, there are no simple answers yet, but watching your calorie and fat intake and getting regular exercise can help. If the medication causes increased sensitivity to the sun, use suntan lotion with a sun protection factor of at least 15 whenever out in the sun.

You and Your Doctor Can Decide How Long You Will Remain on Medication

It may take three weeks to three months to establish the proper dosage of one of these medications. After symptoms are under control, your physician should suggest when you can begin tapering off a medication. This could be from several weeks to twelve to eighteen months (or even not at all), depending on the conditions. Throughout this time, you should actively face your anxiety-provoking situations, using skills similar to those described in this book. As you taper off the medications, you may experience some return of your symptoms. Be patient as your body adjusts to being medication-free, and continue to practice your skills. After about one month, you and your doctor will be able to assess how well you are handling the stresses of your life without medication. If needed, you can discuss a return to that medication or some alternative drug. If you and your doctor decide that long-term use of the medication is the best alternative for you, the physician will help you reduce the medicine to the lowest possible dose that controls the symptoms.

Gradually Taper These Medications

Once you begin treatment with one of these medications, you should never abruptly discontinue your daily dose. Your prescribing physician will direct you in a safe withdrawal process, which may take several days to several months, depending on the condition.

Medications Are Optional

You always have a choice regarding the use of medication. Do not let anyone persuade you that you must take drugs as your only option to overcome an anxiety disorder, or that they offer the only cure for anxiety symptoms. As you have read throughout this book, many forces come to bear on your anxiety. Symptoms can reflect any one of several different psychological disorders and many physical problems. Keep your mind open to all your options in resolving this difficulty. If you choose to use medications as part of your treatment, do so because of your values and beliefs and your trust in your physician. We know from research and clinical experience that these medications are of no benefit to some people and can make matters worse for others. If medications do not benefit you, continue to give other options a fair trial.

Are You Dependent on Drugs or Alcohol?

About 24 percent of people with a long-standing anxiety disorder also have difficulty with drug or alcohol abuse. If you are having this kind of trouble, it is best to get treatment for your chemical dependency while you develop skills to cope with your anxiety. Consider participating in a long-term recovery program such as Alcoholics Anonymous (AA) or Narcotics Anonymous (NA). Stopping your drug or alcohol dependency will give you a much better chance of achieving your goals of recovering from your anxiety problems. It is also most important that you inform your prescribing physician that you are currently having trouble with drug use, or if you have in the past. That will help your doctor determine which of your symptoms relate directly to anxiety and will help him or her to choose the right medication for you. For instance, antidepressants or buspirone are usually better choices for anxious patients who have been chemically dependent because they do not lead to dependency or abuse.

Handling Sexual Side Effects

Some SSRI medications can cause sexual side effects such as reduction in desire or arousal or the inability to have an orgasm. There are several options to respond to this problem if you are taking an SSRI.

1. *The wait-and-see approach.* For some people, these unwanted side effects will diminish and satisfactory sexual functioning will return after the initial several weeks of treatment.

2. *Decrease the dosage.* If the symptoms do not diminish, your doctor may lower your dose of medication to find the minimum effective level for your anxiety. However, you must measure the reduction of your sexual side effects against any diminished ability of the lower-dose medication to treat your primary complaints, or to prevent a relapse of your anxious symptoms.

3. *Take a drug holiday.* It may be possible to take a break from your medication for one to three days or even longer. This could enable you to increase your sexual function during that time. Keep in mind that the SSRI fluoxetine remains in the system too long for a drug holiday to be effective.

4. *Change medication.* Your doctor may suggest that you try a different medication that could have less sexual side effects.

Add a medication. It is possible that adding a medication to the SSRI will help this problem. Drugs that have been used for this purpose include: amantadine (Symmetrel), dextroamphetamine (Dexedrine), methylphenidate (Ritalin), permoline (Cylert), cyproheptadine (Periactin), buspirone (BuSpar), bupropion (Wellbutrin), nefazodone (Serzone), mirtazapine (Remeron), yohimbine (Aphrodyne), granisetron (Kytril), and sildenafil (Viagra).

Medications During Pregnancy

The benzodiazepines are never to be used while attempting to become pregnant, during pregnancy, or while breastfeeding.

Information available on the safety of antidepressant use during pregnancy is limited by the small size and the designs of most trials. However, there is growing evidence that taking selective serotonin reuptake inhibitors (SSRIs) and other related antidepressants during pregnancy carries an extra risk. For this reason, the American College of Obstetricians and Gynecologists

(ACOG) recommends against their use during pregnancy unless it is absolutely required and no other options exist. SSRIs have been found to cause SSRI neonatal withdrawal syndrome and SSRI abstinence syndrome, as well as an increased risk for birth defects. About one out of three newborn infants exposed to antidepressants in the womb shows signs of neonatal drug withdrawal, including tremors, gastrointestinal problems, muscle tensing, sleep disturbances, and high-pitched crying. Other complications from SSRIs or selective norepinephrine reuptake inhibitors (SNRIs) can include irritability, difficulty feeding, and rapid breathing. Studies have found that one particular SSRI, if used during the first trimester, may increase the risk of congenital cardiac malformations. In addition, for every one hundred women taking an SSRI medication late in pregnancy, one may have a child with persistent pulmonary hypertension (PPHN).

At the same time, the symptoms of anxiety disorders and depression can have their own effects on the health of the mother and the fetus. The decision to use or not to use medication during pregnancy and during breast feeding is an important one.

Medication Profiles

You will find a list of all the specific medications within each category on the chart at the end of this chapter.

Selective Serotonin Reuptake Inhibitors (SSRIs)

SSRIs primarily assist the brain in maintaining an increased supply of the neurotransmitter serotonin. Researchers associate a deficiency of serotonin with depression and obsessive-compulsive disorder and implicate it in panic disorder and other psychological problems.

- *Possible benefits.* SSRIs can be helpful for depression, panic disorder, social anxiety, obsessive-compulsive disorder, generalized anxiety, and PTSD. They are well tolerated medications that are safe for medically ill or frail patients and safe in overdose. There are no withdrawal effects unless the patient stops them abruptly, and no dependency develops. They generally do not promote weight gain.

- *Possible disadvantages.* It takes four to six weeks to notice significant therapeutic benefits from the SSRIs. The full range of benefits can take twelve weeks. Patients often experience a temporary worsening of anxiety symptoms during the first two weeks of treatment. SSRIs cause sexual problems more than other antidepressants or benzodiazepines. In fact, this may be their principal limitation, occurring in as many as 35 to 40 percent of patients. It is unclear whether these problems are evident in one SSRI more than others. Abrupt discontinuation of this class of drugs could cause flulike symptoms.
- *Possible side effects.* Nausea, insomnia, headaches, sexual difficulties, initial agitation.

Serotonin-Norepinephrine Reuptake Inhibitors (SNRIs)

Two SNRIs show some benefits for anxiety disorders. I have detailed them separately since there are a few significant differences.

Venlafaxine-XR (Effexor-XR)

Possible benefits. Helpful for panic, obsessive-compulsive disorder, social anxiety disorder, generalized anxiety, and depression.

Possible disadvantages. Takes several weeks for primary effects to begin. Nausea and dizziness can be common side effects. Use during pregnancy or while breast-feeding only after approval from your physician.

Possible side effects. Headache, drowsiness, dizziness, nervousness, trouble sleeping, dry mouth, nausea, vomiting, blurred vision, altered taste, sweating, stomach upset, constipation, loss of appetite, anxiety, or yawning may occur. Increased blood pressure at high doses.

Duloxetine (Cymbalta)

Possible benefits. Helpful for depression, generalized anxiety, panic, OCD.

Possible disadvantages. Therapeutic response can take four to six weeks. Avoid alcohol. Consult your physician regarding use during pregnancy or while breast-feeding.

Possible side effects. Anorexia, constipation, diarrhea, dizziness, drowsiness, fatigue, sweating, insomnia, nausea, dry mouth, reduced libido.

Benzodiazepines (BZs)

- *Possible benefits.* You can take benzodiazepines as a single-dose therapy or several times a day for months (or even years). They are quick-acting. Tolerance does not develop in the anti-panic or other therapeutic effects. Overdose is not dangerous.
- *Possible side effects.* Some patients experience the sedative effects of drowsiness or lethargy, decreased mental sharpness, slurring of speech, and some decrease in co-ordination or unsteadiness of gait, less occupational efficiency or productivity and, occasionally, headache. These may continue during the first few weeks, but tend to clear up, especially if you increase the dose gradually. Sexual side effects can arise. Some people experience low moods, irritability, or agitation. Rarely, some patients will experience disinhibition: they lose control of some of their impulses and do things they wouldn't ordinarily do, like increased arguing, driving the car recklessly, or shoplifting. BZs also increase the effects of alcohol. A patient taking a BZ should drink

very little alcohol and should refrain from drinking within hours of driving a car.

If taken over long periods, the BZs can produce a loss of muscle coordination and some cognitive impairment, especially in the elderly.

- *Disadvantages with BZs.* There are two primary disadvantages with BZs. The first is *abuse potential.* Although it is rare for a person with an anxiety disorder to abuse a benzodiazepine, more patients with a history of substance abuse report a euphoric effect from the BZs than do control subjects. They also can use the BZs to help with sleep, to control anxiety produced by other drugs, or to reduce withdrawal symptoms from other drugs. Because of these concerns, it may not be in the best interest of patients who have both panic disorder and a current substance abuse problem to use the BZs for their anxiety.

  The second disadvantage is that there can be symptoms upon tapering off. Studies indicate that 35 to 45 percent of patients are able to withdraw from the BZs without difficulty. With the others, three different problems can arise: withdrawal, relapse, and rebound. These can sometimes occur simultaneously.

- *Dependence and withdrawal symptoms.* Physical dependence means that when a person stops taking a drug or reduces the dose quickly, he or she will experience symptoms of withdrawal. BZ withdrawal symptoms usually begin soon after reduction of the drug begins. They can be any of the following: confusion, diarrhea, blurred vision, heightened sensory perception, muscle cramping, reduced sensation of smell, muscle twitches, numbness or tingling, decreased appetite, and weight loss. These symptoms can be bothersome but are usually mild to moderate, almost never dangerous, and resolve over the period of a week or so.

At least 50 percent of patients experience some withdrawal symptoms when they stop taking a benzo-diazepine, and almost all patients experience strong withdrawal symptoms if they stop the medication suddenly. Most experts recommend tapering off quite slowly, often taking months to completely discontinue the benzodiazepine.

A higher dosage of a BZ, as well as longer use, can increase the intensity and frequency of the withdrawal symptoms. Short-acting drugs (Xanax, Serax, Ativan) are more likely to produce withdrawal reactions than longer-lasting BZs (Valium, Librium, Tranxene) if they are discontinued rapidly, although the difference is usually small if they are tapered off in an appropriately slow manner. Panic patients seem to be more susceptible to withdrawal symptoms than those with other anxiety disorders.

- *Relapse symptoms*. Relapse means your original anxiety symptoms return after you reduce or stop the medication. Often in relapse the symptoms are not as severe or as frequent as they were before treatment began. Withdrawal symptoms start as the medication is reduced and end one to two weeks after stopping a medication. If the symptoms persist four to six weeks after complete withdrawal, it probably indicates relapse.
- *Rebound symptoms*. Rebound is the temporary return of greater anxiety symptoms after withdrawal from medication than you experienced before the medication. This usually occurs two to three days after a taper and is often caused by too big of a reduction of the drug at one time. It is possible that a rebound reaction can trigger a relapse reaction. Between 10 and 35 percent of patients will experience the rebound of anxiety symptoms, especially panic attacks, when they discontinue the BZs too rapidly.
- A *slow tapering* of the medication is best. One approach

is to remain at each new lower dose for two weeks before the next reduction. Tapering a BZ over a two- to four-month period can lead to significantly fewer withdrawal symptoms.

Possible Symptoms of Withdrawal from Benzodiazepines

Nervousness
Insomnia
Decreased appetite
Blurred vision
Headache
Perspiration
Muscle aches, cramping, or twitching
Altered sensory perception
  (i.e., noises sound very loud, metallic taste, reduced sense of smell)

Poor concentration
Confusion
Diarrhea
Numbness or tingling
Lack of coordination
Lack of energy

An additional problem associated with BZs is connected with alcohol use. Alcohol will increase the drug's depressant effects on the brain and can result in excessive drowsiness or intoxication.

Benzodiazepines should never be taken while attempting to become pregnant, while pregnant, or while breast-feeding.

Tricyclic Antidepressants (TCAs)

Physicians use tricyclic antidepressants in the treatment of panic disorder, PTSD, generalized anxiety, and depression that occurs with anxiety. Of this family, imipramine has been the focus of most of the panic treatment research.

- *Possible benefits.* Often effective in reducing panic attacks and elevating depressed mood. Well researched. Usually a single daily dose. Tolerance does not develop. Nonaddicting.

- *Possible disadvantages.* Onset takes four to twelve weeks. Possible side effects initially (including insomnia, tremor, or both) may last up to the first two to three weeks of treatment. Weight gain can be as much as one pound per month with about 25 percent of patients gaining twenty pounds or more. Dangerous in overdose. Should not be used by patients with narrow-angle glaucoma or certain heart abnormalities. Men with an enlarged prostate should avoid certain antidepressants.
- *Possible side effects.* The anticholinergic effects of dry mouth, blurred vision, constipation, and difficulty in urination; postural hypotension; tachycardia; loss of sex drive; erectile failure; increased sensitivity to the sun; weight gain; sedation (sleepiness); increased sweating. Some side effects will disappear with the passage of time or with a decrease in the dosage. Some people may experience side effects such as jitteriness, irritation, unusual energy, and difficulty falling or staying asleep on dosages as low as 10 mg per day.
- *Dosages recommended by investigators.* One-third of panic-prone individuals become jittery and actually experience more anxiety symptoms for the first two to three weeks. For this reason, the medication trial should probably be initiated with a very low dose—as little as 10 to 25 milligrams (mg) per day of imipramine, for example. If uncomfortable side effects appear, one approach is to wait two to three weeks for them to diminish before increasing to the next higher dose. If the patient adjusts to the side effects, the physician increases the dosage every two or more days until the patient is taking the preferred dosage.

If daytime sedation or other side effects are bothersome to the patient, the physician may suggest taking the full dosage at night before bedtime.

- *Tapering.* Your doctor may suggest that you begin to taper your TCA six months to a year after you have controlled your panic attacks. You can taper it gradually over a two- to three-week period to avoid the flu-like symptoms that commonly occur if you abruptly stop the medication. Even more gradual tapering can help monitor for a relapse in panic attacks. If you stop this medication abruptly, withdrawal symptoms may begin within twenty-four hours, including nausea, tremor, headache, and insomnia. Few symptoms should be evident with a gradual decrease in dose. Panic attacks will not usually return immediately after you stop the medication, but may recur several weeks later.

Monoamine Oxidase Inhibitors (MAOIs)

Monoamine oxidase inhibitors, commonly called MAOIs, are the other major antidepressant family. Phenelzine (Nardil) is the MAOI most researched for the treatment of panic. Another that may be effective against panic attacks is tranylcypromine (Parnate).

- *Possible benefits.* Helpful in reducing panic attacks, elevating depressed mood, and increasing confidence. Can also help OCD, generalized anxiety, PTSD, and social anxiety. Well studied. Tolerance does not develop. Non-addicting.
- *Possible disadvantages.* Dietary and medication restrictions are important and can be bothersome to some people. These include avoiding certain foods like aged cheese or meat and certain medications like cold remedies. Some agitation during first days. Requires weeks to months for full therapeutic effects. Not as helpful for anticipatory anxiety. Dangerous in overdose.
- *Dietary restrictions.* Certain foods contain a substance called tyramine, which, when combined with an MAOI,

can cause a "hypertensive crisis" that can produce dangerously high blood pressure, a severe headache, stiff neck, nausea, or stroke.

The patient using an MAOI must be responsible, since this medication requires significant dietary restrictions. To be avoided are: cheese (except cottage, farmer, or cream cheese), sour cream, homemade yogurt, red wine, vermouth, liquors, beer, ale, sherry, cognac, Bovril and Marmite yeast extracts (baked goods prepared with yeast are OK), aged meats and fish, meat prepared with tenderizer, liver and liverwurst, overripe bananas, fava beans, Italian green beans, Chinese and English pea pods, and lima beans.

Foods to eat in moderation include avocados, chocolate, figs, raisins and dates, soy sauce, caffeinated drinks, white wine, and distilled alcoholic beverages (whiskey, gin, vodka).

- *Medication restrictions.* MAOIs have major interactions with many other drugs, including anesthetics, analgesics, other antidepressants, and anxiolytics. The patient using an MAOI should always consult the prescribing physician before taking any additional medications. This especially includes over-the-counter cold medicines (including nose drops or sprays), amphetamines, diet pills, tricyclic antidepressants, and certain antihistamines.
- *Possible side effects.* Difficulty sleeping; increased appetite; sexual side effects, especially difficulty achieving orgasms for men and women; weight gain; dry mouth; sedation (sleepiness); and low blood pressure symptoms, particularly on standing up rapidly, which can lead to postural hypotension.

As with any antidepressant, some patients will experience hypomania, which causes them to feel unusually "high" and full of energy, talkative, and very self-confident, with little need for sleep, and a high sex drive. Patients don't always recognize this as a problem, but it can certainly be irritating to those around them and should be reported to the prescribing physician.

Beta-Blockers

Beta-blockers can be helpful in the treatment of the physical symptoms of anxiety, especially social anxiety. Physicians prescribe them to control rapid heartbeat, shaking, trembling, and blushing in anxious situations for several hours.

- *Possible benefits.* Safe for most patients. Few side effects. Not habit-forming.
- *Possible disadvantages.* Often social anxiety symptoms are so strong that beta-blockers, while helpful, cannot reduce enough of the symptoms to provide relief. Because they can lower blood pressure and slow heart rate, people diagnosed with low blood pressure or heart conditions may not be able to take them. Not recommended for patients with asthma or any other respiratory illness that causes wheezing or for patients with diabetes.

Other Tranquilizers

Buspirone (BuSpar)

Possible benefits. Buspirone is helpful for generalized anxiety, OCD, and panic. Much less likely to cause drowsiness and fatigue than the benzodiazepines. A very safe medication. It is not habit-forming, and there are no withdrawal symptoms.

Possible disadvantages. Unlike the benzodiazepines, buspirone does not work right away. You can't take one as needed and expect to notice benefits. Avoid use during first three months of pregnancy. Consult physician regarding use in last six months of pregnancy or while breast-feeding.

Possible side effects. Few. Headache and dizziness can each occur in 3 to 12 percent of patients, but usually go away in a few days. Mild drowsiness is possible.

Anticonvulsants

Gabapentin (Neurontin)
Possible benefits. May be useful for social anxiety and generalized anxiety disorder. May work better by adding it to a primary medication that is not completely effective.

Possible disadvantages. Consult a physician before use during pregnancy or while breast-feeding.

Possible side effects. Dizziness, dry mouth, drowsiness, nausea, flatulence, and decreased libido.

Valproic Acid (Depakote)
Possible benefits. Valproic acid is an epilepsy medication that is now used for the treatment of panic attacks as well as other psychiatric problems. May work better by adding it to a primary medication that is not completely effective.

Possible disadvantages. Can cause bruising or bleeding when taken with aspirin. Can cause excessive sedation (sleepiness) with alcohol and also with Klonopin or other benzodiazepines. Can cause liver problems. To monitor your liver function and your platelet count, your doctor may ask you to take a simple blood test every two months for the first six months and every three to four months after that. Avoid using during pregnancy and while breast-feeding.

Possible side effects. Valproic acid is well tolerated. Nausea, vomiting, indigestion, headache, confusion, and drowsiness sometimes occur but usually subside in a few weeks.

Medications for Anxiety Disorders

Medication	Used in Treatment of
Benzodiazepines	
alprazolam (Xanax)	panic[†], generalized anxiety, phobias, social anxiety, OCD
clonazepam (Klonopin)	panic[†], generalized anxiety, phobias, social anxiety
diazepam (Valium)	panic, generalized anxiety, phobias
lorazepam (Ativan)	panic, generalized anxiety, phobias
oxazepam (Serax)	generalized anxiety, phobias
chlordiazepoxide (Librium)	generalized anxiety, phobias
Selective Serotonin Reuptake Inhibitors (SSRIs)	
fluoxetine (Prozac)	panic[†], OCD[†], social anxiety, generalized anxiety, PTSD
fluvoxamine (Luvox)	panic, OCD[†], social anxiety, generalized anxiety, PTSD
sertraline (Zoloft)	panic[†], OCD[†], social anxiety[†], PTSD[†], generalized anxiety
paroxetine (Paxil)	panic[†], OCD[†], social anxiety[†], generalized anxiety[†], PTSD[†]
escitalopram oxalate (Lexapro)	panic, OCD, social anxiety, generalized anxiety, PTSD
citalopram (Celexa)	panic, OCD, social anxiety, generalized anxiety, PTSD
Serotonin-Norepinephrine Reuptake Inhibitors (SNRIs)	
venlafaxine (Effexor)	panic[†], social anxiety, generalized anxiety, OCD
venlafaxine XR (Effexor XR)	panic[†], social anxiety[†], generalized anxiety[†], OCD
duloxetine (Cymbalta)	generalized anxiety[†], social anxiety, panic, OCD

[†]=approved by the FDA for treatment of this disorder.

(continued on next page)

Medications for Anxiety Disorders *(continued)*

Medication	Used in Treatment of
Tricyclic Antidepressants	
imipramine (Tofranil)	panic, generalized anxiety, PTSD
desipramine (Norpramin & others)	panic, generalized anxiety, PTSD
nortriptyline (Aventyl or Pamelor)	panic, generalized anxiety, PTSD
amitriptyline (Elavil)	panic, generalized anxiety, PTSD
doxepin (Sinequan or Adapin)	panic
clomipramine (Anafranil)	OCD†, panic
Other Antidepressant	
trazodone (Desyrel)	panic, generalized anxiety
Monoamine Oxidase Inhibitors (MAOIs)	
phenelzine (Nardil)	panic, OCD, generalized anxiety, social anxiety, PTSD
tranylcypromine (Parnate)	panic, OCD, generalized anxiety, PTSD
Beta-Blockers	
propranolol (Inderal)	social anxiety
atenolol (Tenormin)	social anxiety
Mild Tranquilizer	
buspirone (BuSpar)	generalized anxiety†, panic, OCD
Anticonvulsants	
valproate (Depakote)	panic
pregabalin (Lyrica)	generalized anxiety disorder
gabapentin (Neurontin)	generalized anxiety disorder, social anxiety

†=approved by the FDA for treatment of this disorder.

Resources

When you go to www.dontpaniclive.com, you will find lots of help, including:

- How to print extra copies of all the practice forms in this book
- How to print free transcripts to create your own recordings for practicing breathing skills and relaxation
- How to order prerecorded CDs of the breathing and relaxation practices
- A free e-newsletter to keep you up-to-date on the latest research on anxiety, as well as new ideas I'm developing about anxiety self-help
- Free online self-help programs for those with panic disorder, fear of flying, obsessive-compulsive disorder, social anxiety, worries, and specific phobias
- Free information on the current medications for anxiety disorders, including recommended dosages, advantages, disadvantages, and side effects
- A list of the other books and kits I have developed for anxiety self-help

E-mail me at rrw@med.unc.edu if you want:

- Help finding a mental health professional near you who specializes in anxiety treatment
- Dates of my two-day treatment programs

Index